Contributors

CONSULTING EDITOR

GREGORY T. CARTER, MD, MS
Consulting Medical Editor, Medical Director, St Luke's Rehabilitation Institute, Spokane, Washington

EDITOR

ROBERT H. MEIER III, MD
Director, Amputee Services of America, Denver, Colorado; Adjunct Faculty, J. E. Hanger College of Orthotics and Prosthetics, St. Petersburg College, St. Petersburg, Florida

AUTHORS

HOWARD P. BELON, PhD
Member of Colorado Psychological Association, Member of the American Psychological Association, Program Psychologist and Licensed Clinical Psychologist, Amputee Services of America, Denver, Colorado

INGER BRUECKNER, PT
Presbyterian/St. Luke's Medical Center, Denver, Colorado

LAURI CONNELLY, OTR/L
Center for Rehabilitation Outcomes Research, Rehabilitation Institute of Chicago, Chicago, Illinois

TIMOTHY R. DILLINGHAM, MD, MS
William J. Erdman, II, Professor and Chair of Physical Medicine and Rehabilitation, Perelman School of Medicine at the University of Pennsylvania, Philadelphia, Pennsylvania

LINDA EHRLICH-JONES, PhD, RN
Center for Rehabilitation Outcomes Research, Rehabilitation Institute of Chicago; Research Assistant Professor, Department of Physical Medicine and Rehabilitation, Feinberg School of Medicine, Northwestern University, Chicago, Illinois

ALBERTO ESQUENAZI, MD
Chair and Professor of Physical Medicine and Rehabilitation and Director, Gait and Motion Analysis Laboratory, MossRehab, Elkins Park, Pennsylvania

STEFANIA FATONE, PhD, BPO (Hon)
Associate Professor, Department of Physical Medicine and Rehabilitation, Feinberg School of Medicine, Northwestern University, Chicago, Illinois

GEORGE C. GONDO, MA
Director, Research and Grants, The Amputee Coalition, Manassas, Virginia

JEFFREY T. HECKMAN, DO
Assistant Professor, Department of Rehabilitation Medicine, University of Washington; Medical Director, Regional Amputation Center (RAC), VA Puget Sound Health Care System, Seattle Division, Seattle, Washington

ALLEN W. HEINEMANN, PhD
Center for Rehabilitation Outcomes Research, Rehabilitation Institute of Chicago; Department of Physical Medicine and Rehabilitation, Feinberg School of Medicine, Northwestern University, Chicago, Illinois

SHAWN SWANSON JOHNSON, BS, OTR/L
Consultant and Independent Contractor, Occupational Therapy, Houston, Texas

ROBERT S. KISTENBERG, MPH, L/CP, FAAOP
Georgia Institute of Technology, School of Applied Physiology, Atlanta, Georgia

JULIE KLARICH, OTR, CHT
Occupational Therapist, Presbyterian/St. Luke's Medical Center, Denver, Colorado

ELIZABETH MANSFIELD, BA
Clinical Education Concepts, Baiting Hollow, New York

ROBERT H. MEIER III, MD
Director, Amputee Services of America, Denver, Colorado Adjunct Faculty, J. E. Hanger College of Orthotics and Prosthetics, St. Petersburg College, St. Petersburg, Florida

DANIELLE MELTON, MD
Director, Amputee Program, TIRR/Memorial Hermann Hospital; Assistant Professor, Departments of Physical Medicine and Rehabilitation and Orthopedic Surgery, University of Texas Medical School, Houston, Texas

THOMAS PASSERO, AS, CP
American Board for Certification in Orthotics and Prosthetics, Graduate, Prosthetic and Orthotic Program, Northwestern University Medical School; Clinical Director, Prosthetic and Orthotic Associates, Inc, Handspring Upper Limb Prosthetic Specialists, Middletown, New York

DAVID SCHNUR, MD
Plastic Surgery Clinic of Denver, Denver, Colorado

TERRENCE PATRICK SHEEHAN, MD
Chief Medical Officer, Adventist Rehabilitation Hospital of Maryland, Rockville, Maryland; Medical Director, Amputee Coalition of America, Manassas, Virginia

MARGARET G. STINEMAN, MD
Professor, Physical Medicine and Rehabilitation and Epidemiology, Department of Physical Medicine and Rehabilitation, Center for Clinical Epidemiology and Biostatistics, Perelman School of Medicine at the University of Pennsylvania, Philadelphia, Pennsylvania

HEIKKI UUSTAL, MD
JFK-Johnson Rehab Institute, Edison; Associate Professor, Physical Medicine and Rehabilitation, Rutgers-Robert Wood Johnson Medical School, Piscataway, New Jersey

PRIYA VARMA, MD, MPH
Resident, Department of Physical Medicine and Rehabilitation, Perelman School of Medicine at the University of Pennsylvania, Philadelphia, Pennsylvania

DIANE F. VIGODA, LCSW, CCM
Member of Colorado Chapter of The National Association of Social Workers, Certified
Case Manager through The Commission for Case Manager Certification, Team Leader
and Counselor, Amputee Services of America, Denver, Colorado

STANLEY YOO, MD
Moss Rehab, Elkins Park, Pennsylvania

Contents

In 2005, 1.6 million people were estimated to be living with limb loss; by 2050, the rate is expected to double to 3.6 million in the United States. Past data have shown that the rates of dysvascular amputations were increasing. However, recent studies looking at single diseases of peripheral arterial disease and diabetes mellitus show amputations related to these conditions are now decreasing. The authors think that it may not be a single disease process but rather the cumulative illness burden that is leading to amputations. In addition to cause, age, gender, and race continue to play a role in limb loss.

The amputee gets lost in the American health care system because of fragmentation across the continuum. The journey of the diabetic patient with limb loss through the health care system is even more precarious than that of the traumatic amputee. Interventions to address these secondary conditions and improve the health and outcomes of persons with disability have focused on standard medical treatments, such as medication or physical rehabilitation therapies, often to the exclusion of psychosocial interventions. Each member of the amputee rehabilitation team plays a specific and important role in the care and recovery of the person with limb loss.

Providing rehabilitation services for the person with an amputation has become more difficult in today's health care environment. Amputation rehabilitation calls for specialized, multidisciplinary rehabilitation training. In examining the principles of amputation rehabilitation, one must understand the lessons learned from the Veterans Affairs Amputation System of Care and return to the founding principles of rehabilitation medicine. Persons with amputations must be reevaluated in a tight program of follow-up care.

The best level of amputation must take into consideration the newest socket designs, methods of prosthetic suspension, and technologically advanced components. In some instances stump revision should be considered, to provide a better prosthetic fitting and function. Targeted reinnervation is a new neural-machine interface that has been developed to help improve the function of electrically powered upper prosthetic limbs. Osseointegrated implants for prosthetic suspension offer amputees an alternative to the traditional socket suspension, and are especially useful for transfemoral and transhumeral levels of amputation. Cadaver bone can be used to lengthen an extremely short residual bony lever arm.

Most people with amputations should not experience pain that interferes with their quality of life or requires regular medication more than 6 months following the amputation surgery. In fact, most people with amputations do not experience significant pain more than 3 months following the amputation. However, the clinician must specifically define what these patients mean when they relate that they have pain. The pain must be carefully differentiated to treat it properly. Most problematic pain that is present more than 6 months after amputation is related to a poorly fitting prosthesis and should be labeled as residual limb pain.

Individuals experience multiple changes as a result of amputation. These changes not only are physical in nature but also may include psychological, financial, and comfort changes across the spectrum of an individual's life. It is important to assess the emotional responses that an individual may experience postsurgery and throughout the rehabilitation process. Grieving is a natural and normal emotional response postamputation. Grief resolution is one of the primary areas of focus in counseling amputees. This article examines various factors and strategies used in the adaptation and recovery from amputation.

This article reviews occupational therapy treatment and physical therapy treatment during preprosthetic training for upper and lower extremity amputees. Review of preoperative intervention, preparing the residual limb for the prosthesis, instruction in techniques, and adaptive equipment for activities of daily living, as well as suggestions for return to vocational and avocational activities are addressed.

by 2050 to 3.6 million, making an understanding of management of the individual with amputation essential for the physiatrist. This article highlights common complications following amputation and discusses the approach to evaluation, treatment, and developing management strategies to ensure optimal functional outcomes for this population of patients.

Outcome measurement is crucial to assuring high-quality patient services and improving the quality of services provided by prosthetists. This article summarizes recent evidence on the measurement properties of outcome measures, and updates previously published summaries of outcome instruments. The review focuses on measures of mobility, functional status, quality of life, and patient satisfaction, and includes both performance-based and patient-reported outcomes. Amputation-specific and general measures that are suitable for patients served by prosthetists are discussed. It is encouraging that responsiveness of measures is often reported, as this information is needed to improve clinical utility.

This article provides a generalized overview of amputation classifications and the idealized outcomes for upper and lower amputations at their respective levels. The following levels are discussed: above knee/transfemoral, below knee/transtibial, above elbow/transhumeral, below elbow/transradial, and bilateral for upper and lower extremities. This classification defines a framework for clinicians to share with patients so that they understand the potential for their expected functional outcomes regarding mobility and activities of daily living, both with and without a prosthesis. Moreover, it addresses some of the vocational and avocational needs of the individual regarding amputation.

PHYSICAL MEDICINE & REHABILITATION CLINICS OF NORTH AMERICA

RELATED INTEREST

Hand Clinics, November 2011
Hand Transplantation
Gerald Brandacher, MD, and W.P. Andrew Lee, MD, *Editors*

VISIT THE CLINICS ONLINE!
Access your subscription at:
www.theclinics.com

**DOWNLOAD
Free App!**

**Review Articles
THE CLINICS**

NOW AVAILABLE FOR YOUR iPhone and iPad

Foreword

Contemporary Amputee Rehabilitation

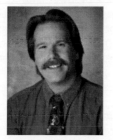

Gregory T. Carter, MD, MS
Consulting Editor

This volume is guest edited by my long-time close friend, Dr Robert H. "Skip" Meier III. I first met Dr Meier when I was a resident physician in Sacramento, CA. Dr Meier would come out periodically to teach us the principles of amputee rehabilitation. It is my distinct pleasure to write the foreword for this volume guest edited by Dr Meier covering this important topic, which has become so important now with many of our wounded veterans returning from service in the Middle East. I know of no one more skilled in the area of amputee rehabilitation than Dr Meier, and he has assembled a very distinguished group of authors to help write this edition of *Physical Medicine and Rehabilitation Clinics of North America*.

Dr Meier has worked with thousands of adults and children who have sustained an amputation of one or more limbs in his career, which now spans over 40 years. This includes services he has volunteered for, such as working with victims of land mine injuries in warring countries overseas. Dr Meier has truly dedicated his entire career to this field.

One of the authors recruited by Dr Meier is the chairman and Chief Medical Officer of Moss Rehabilitation, Dr Alberto Esquenazi. Dr Esquenazi is himself an amputee due to an accident incurred while he was still in medical school. Dr Meier was Dr Esquenazi's first rehabilitation physician following his limb loss. Dr Esquenazi later wrote the book on field amputation for the World Health Organization and has gone on to a brilliant academic career himself.

Both Dr Meier and Dr Esquenazi emphasize getting amputees back into life as fully and meaningfully as possible. The basis of achieving these types of positive results comes from a deep understanding of the patient's personal goals and their relationships to family, friends, and community that existed prior to the amputation.

Among the other esteemed authors is my friend and colleague, Dr Tim Dillingham. Dr Dillingham is currently the chair of the Department of Physical Medicine and Rehabilitation at the University of Pennsylvania and Chief Medical Officer for Good

Phys Med Rehabil Clin N Am 25 (2014) xiii–xiv
http://dx.doi.org/10.1016/j.pmr.2013.10.002
1047-9651/14/$ – see front matter

Shepherd Penn Partners. Dr Dillingham brings a vast wealth of knowledge to this project as well, including particular expertise in the etiology and changing demographics of amputation in our world today. Dr Dillingham has published extensively in the area of methodology to improve outcomes for persons with amputations in both acute and postacute settings.

Dr Terrence P. Sheehan, a physiatrist and medical director of Kessler-Adventist Rehabilitation Hospital, brings his expertise regarding the effects of lower limb loss on patients. Dr Sheehan has researched back and hip problems caused by the stress and strain of walking with an improper gait, using prostheses, or using crutches. This can sometimes be more of a problem for lower extremity amputees than phantom pain. Dr Sheehan's work has helped document that lower-extremity amputation causes a change in the center of gravity, disrupting the biomechanical symmetry of the back and hips. Thus, the muscles and joints of the low back are subject to greater stress, leading to chronic pain.

Drs Uustal and Yoo bring extensive knowledge of prosthetic rehabilitation issues in the diabetic and dysvascular amputee population. Their past work has documented the importance of evaluation and management of diabetic and dysvascular patients with lower limb from the preprosthetic phase all the way through until final prosthetic fitting.

Dr Vigoda and Belon discuss the emotional adjustment to limb loss, which has been a major problem given the nature of injuries our troops have suffered during the conflicts in Iraq and Afghanistan.

Robert S. Kistenberg, MPH, CP, from the School of Applied Physiology at Georgia Technical University, brings extensive expertise on activation in motor-related cortical areas on viewing limb movements and how that may be used to help prosthesis users imitate movements of other prosthesis users to help with motor planning. This has significant implications on how amputee rehabilitation is done and suggests that involving another experienced prosthesis user may help with the adaptive learning process.

I also want to thank all the other distinguished authors, including Drs Varma, Passero, Swanson-Johnson, Heinemann and Ms Karich and Ms Brueckner, for their contributions to this issue of *Physical Medicine and Rehabilitation Clinics of North America*. It is truly a comprehensive presentation of management of the amputee patient and provides real-life useful recommendations on how to resolve the myriad of problems they can present with. The contributions of these authors to this issue give us a remarkably useful addition to the *Physical Medicine and Rehabilitation Clinics of North America* series.

Gregory T. Carter, MD, MS
Medical Director
St Luke's Rehabilitation Institute
711 South Cowley Street
Spokane, WA 99202, USA

E-mail address:
gtcarter@uw.edu

Preface

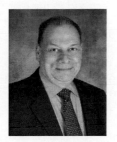

Robert H. Meier III, MD
Editor

I have been involved in the areas of amputation, prosthetics, amputation rehabilitation, outcomes, and emotional issues for persons with amputation since 1969 when I first worked with two Army warrant officer helicopter pilots who had each lost a leg below the knee while flying in Vietnam. They wished to remain on active duty and to fulfill their passion for flying. As a flight surgeon at that time, they had to begin their journey to become certified for flying once again by seeing their local flight surgeon at Ft. Eustis, Virginia. That flight surgeon happened to be me. Both of these men persisted, completed all their tests, and passed their in-flight examination to become certified pilots once again. To both of these men, Bruce McQuilken and Mike Pignataro, I owe my professional career as a rehabilitation physician. They were the starting point to my many experiences in working with persons who have lost some part of their bodies, yet have returned to fully functional lives and have made significant contributions to their families and communities. Along the way, I have been inspired by giants in the fields of surgery, physiatry, prosthetics, therapy, psychology, outcome studies, and vocational rehabilitation. For, in the comprehensive nature of amputation rehabilitation, it truly does "take a village." One health professional cannot truly provide all of the services essential to obtain the best outcome for the person who sustains an amputation. It does indeed take a dedicated, experienced, and communicative team of professionals who are willing to listen to the amputee who is going through the adaptive process that we call rehabilitation.

However, along my journey and for those of you perhaps over the age of 40 years, we have seen many, many changes in our own fields as well as changes in society, wartime conflict, technologic advances, health care financing, and the struggle for professional autonomy. With the changes in health care financing, we see the emphasis in health care delivery moved from the inpatient rehabilitation hospital to the outpatient setting or the home setting. Can amputation rehabilitation truly be achieved through home health service delivery? The traditional rehabilitation team has been pulled apart and access to traditional rehabilitation services is now restricted by some health care sponsors. We are constantly challenged to find more creative ways to deliver services in a more efficient manner. Yet, we now see new technology with an increased price tag in arm and leg prostheses. Do we have physicians and therapists who understand

Phys Med Rehabil Clin N Am 25 (2014) xv–xvii
http://dx.doi.org/10.1016/j.pmr.2013.10.003
1047-9651/14/$ – see front matter © 2014 Published by Elsevier Inc.

pmr.theclinics.com

how to use these new technologies to their fullest ability? Do we have scientific studies that permit us to choose the most cost-effective prosthetic advances that are matched to the individual person with an amputation? Or, do we respond to the marketing hype and anecdotal feedback from users and manufacturers? In addition, we are in the age of cyber-information. If a new amputee goes online and explores YouTube, they will have access to videos extolling the virtues of the Genium knee, the I-Limb, the Michelangelo hand, or the Biom foot/ankle. While these are new technologies and very sexy for the public, when should they be used and when are they not superior to prior designs that have stood the test of time? As we become more bionically or robotically focused, what is reasonable to prescribe, fabricate, or financially sponsor?

As we have changed from the inpatient setting to an inpatient medical and rehabilitation model, how do we educate, train, and follow the person whose life has changed because of the amputation? Who can legitimately claim a part of the patient pie: the doctor, the prosthetist, the therapist, the case manager, the nurse, the psychologist, or the insurance carrier? Whose interests take priority and can these individuals work together as a cohesive team to achieve the desired outcomes?

While I may be considered an old fogy with outmoded medical practices, there are still many fine principles from earlier days that should be considered in the practice of amputation rehabilitation. While it would seem that in today's culture, amputation rehabilitation is equated to the provision of the prosthesis, it should be so much more than just a focus on the prosthesis. The opportunity for the best functional outcomes, return to a high quality of life, and a positive emotional adaptation to limb loss must be facilitated as a part of a comprehensive and essential array of rehabilitation services.

Persons of my generation grew up with the childhood images of Long John Silver and Captain Hook as the embodiment of the person who wore a peg leg or a hook instead of a hand. These were characters that took on lives that had some negative or even evil personas. Fortunately, while these images are still in childhood tales, we have role models that demonstrate a much more positive personality and lifestyle outcome. I have to thank folks like Aaron Ralston, Hector Picard, Rich Stewart, Steve Hooper, Barbie Thomas, Sean McHugh, Mike Pignataro, Eric Nelson, Tom Passero, Samoana Matagi, Mike St.Onge, Paco Torres, Steve Kinnett, and Albert Esquenazi, who have taught me that there is more to an amputee's life than a prosthetic prescription, a hook, or a peg leg. Sometimes it is a snowboard, a sit ski, a rifle, wiping a bum by yourself, exhibiting extraordinary muscle development, pleasuring a partner, motivating a crowd of able-bodied gawkers, and being able to love and be loved. That despite a change in their body image or function, they have been able to accomplish the things they set out to do, which most of us would have felt to be improbable or impossible. One thing I quickly learned as a budding physiatrist was that it was unwise to tell the person with a disability that they could not do something they wished to do. They most always proved me to be a pompous ass and that I had no business suggesting what they could and could not accomplish using their own motivation and ingenuity.

Thanks are in order, and I need to express my special thanks to the faculty at Franklin and Marshall College, who instilled in me a lifelong love of learning. Also, to the faculty of the Temple University School of Medicine, who taught me that there is so much more to medicine than laboratory tests and labeling a person with a diagnosis. I truly learned the art of listening between the lines and words that our patients speak to us.

This issue is designed to bring those with an interest in the person with an amputation into the current decade of rehabilitation services. The authors represent most every field of amputation and prosthetic service that is available in the United States today. A special thanks must be extended here to the authors who took their valuable and busy time to write the sage wisdom and information included here. This issue is a tribute to their expertise and chosen professions. Things are changing so quickly that some of the technology discussed here will be outmoded soon. However, I believe that the principles of rehabilitation will remain steady even though they may be practiced or achieved in differing manners. I hope this issue effectively melds the principles of rehabilitation with the contemporary and changing practices of prosthetics and medicine.

Robert H. Meier III, MD
Amputee Services of America
1601 East 19th Avenue, Suite 5100
Denver, CO 80218, USA

E-mail address:
skipdoc3@gmail.com

Dedication

This publication is dedicated to my teachers, mentors, and friends: Dorothea Daniels Glass, MD and Richard Herman, MD. Dr Herman was Chair of the Department of Rehabilitation Medicine during my residency at Temple University School of Medicine in Philadelphia, Pennsylvania from 1971 to 1977. Dr Glass was Director of Residency Training in Physical Medicine and Rehabilitation and Chair of the Department at Temple from 1977 to 1983. It was under their marvelous tutelage that I spent my formative years as a physiatrist.

A teacher affects eternity. He (she) can never tell where his (her) influence stops.
— From Henry Brooks Adams (journalist, historian, academic, and novelist),
1838–1918, from The Education of Henry Adams.

Robert H. Meier III, MD
Amputee Services of America
Denver, CO, USA

E-mail address:
skipdoc3@gmail.com

Phys Med Rehabil Clin N Am 25 (2014) xix
http://dx.doi.org/10.1016/j.pmr.2013.10.004
1047-9651/14/$ – see front matter © 2014 Published by Elsevier Inc.

pmr.theclinics.com

Epidemiology of Limb Loss

Priya Varma, MD, MPH[a], Margaret G. Stineman, MD[b],
Timothy R. Dillingham, MD, MS[c],*

KEYWORDS

- Amputation • Limb loss • Dysvascular • Transfemoral • Transtibial

KEY POINTS

- In 1996, the incidence of amputations most commonly occurred because of vascular conditions and trauma.
- Dysvascular amputation rates were 8 times greater than trauma-related amputation rates in 1996.
- The number of amputations among patients with diabetes is declining, but the number of patients with diabetes is increasing because of early diagnosis.
- The number of amputations among elderly patients with peripheral arterial disease is declining.
- The combined illness burden of multiple comorbidities increases the risk of amputations.
- Males are at a higher risk for dysvascular and trauma-related amputations than females.
- Racial disparities continue to play a role in dysvascular amputation rates with certain groups; African Americans, Hispanic Americans, and Native Americans having the highest rates.
- Trauma- and cancer-related amputations are declining.

Despite advancements in medicine and the emphasis on disease prevention, limb loss continues to be prevalent in our society.[1] In 2005, 1.6 million people were estimated to be living with limb loss; by 2050, the rate is expected to double to 3.6 million in the United States.[1] Limb loss can be subdivided into 2 types, *major and minor limb loss*. Major limb loss is a transhumeral, transradial, transfemoral, or transtibial amputation. Minor limb loss is defined as an amputation of the hand, digits, toes, or at the midfoot level.[2] The incidence of amputations most commonly relates to vascular conditions, trauma, malignancy, and congenital deficiency.[3] Between the 1980s and 1990s, the amputation rates increased among dysvascular patients and declined in trauma and cancer (**Table 1**). Contemporary studies have shown a

Partially supported by grants 2R42HD069067-02 (TRD) and HD042588R01 (MGS).
[a] Department of Physical Medicine and Rehabilitation, University of Pennsylvania, 1800 Lombard Street, 1st floor, Philadelphia, PA 19146, USA; [b] Department of Physical Medicine and Rehabilitation, Center for Clinical Epidemiology and Biostatistics, University of Pennsylvania, 423 Guardian Drive, 904 Blockley Hall, Philadelphia, PA 19104, USA; [c] Department of Physical Medicine and Rehabilitation, Perelman School of Medicine, University of Pennsylvania, 1800 Lombard Street, 1st floor, Philadelphia, PA 19146, USA
* Corresponding author.
E-mail address: timothy.dillingham@uphs.upenn.edu

Phys Med Rehabil Clin N Am 25 (2014) 1–8
http://dx.doi.org/10.1016/j.pmr.2013.09.001
1047-9651/14/$ – see front matter © 2014 Elsevier Inc. All rights reserved.

Table 1
Change in rates of amputations 1988–1997 HCUP[a]

Year	Dysvascular[a]	Trauma[a]	Cancer[a]
1988	38.3	11.37	0.62
1996	46.19	5.86	0.35
Yearly Change	+3.0%	−5.6%	−4.7%
Overall Change	+27.0%	−50.0%	−43.0%

[a] Rates: Per 100,000 live births.
Modified from Dillingham TR, Pezzin L, MacKenzie E. Limb amputation and limb deficiency: epidemiology and recent trends in the United States. South Med J 2002;95(8):877; with permission.

reduction of rates in subsets of those with diabetes and peripheral arterial disease (PAD). The purpose of this review is to highlight the epidemiology of limb loss and current trends.

DYSVASCULAR

Nationally representative hospital discharge data from 1988 to 1996 from the Healthcare Cost and Utilization Project (HCUP) showed that overall, dysvascular-related amputations were increasing as reported by Dillingham, Pezzin, and MacKenzie[3] in 2002. Increased rates were evident in levels associated with considerable functional impairments, such as the foot, transtibial, and transfemoral levels. Incidence rates of dysvascular amputations increased with age in both sexes and racial groups when comparing African Americans with non-African Americans. Men and African Americans underwent amputations at higher rates compared with Women and non-African Americans (**Fig. 1**). The pattern was noted to be markedly higher among African Americans and women older than 85 years. African Americans older than 85 years were 11.7 times more likely than their middle-aged counterparts to undergo a dysvascular amputation. African Americans were also more likely to have amputations at higher levels than whites.[3] A similar effect was noted among women undergoing dysvascular amputations who were older than 85 years, with a relative risk ratio of 12 compared with middle-aged women.[3]

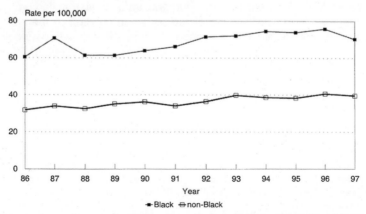

Fig. 1. Age- and gender-standardized rates of dysvascular amputations by race. (*From* Dillingham TR, Pezzin LE, MacKenzie E. Racial differences in the incidence of limb loss secondary to peripheral vascular disease: a population-based study. Arch Phys Med Rehabil 2002;83:1254; with permission.)

DIABETES

Diabetes, a common comorbidity associated with dysvascular disease, affects 25.8 million people.[4] Those patients with diabetes mellitus have an approximately 10-times higher risk of amputation compared with individuals without diabetes.[5] Racial disparities continue to play a role in the course of diabetes. In general, the risk of diagnosed diabetes was 18% higher among Asian Americans, 66% higher among Hispanics, and 77% higher among non-Hispanic blacks compared with non-Hispanic whites.[4] A review by Dillingham, Pezzin, and MacKenzie[6] revealed that research has shown that among those individuals with diabetes, African Americans, Hispanics, and Native Americans are at a considerably higher risk for lower-limb loss than white people.

One objective of Healthy People 2010 was to decrease the rate of lower-extremity amputations among those individuals with diabetes.[7] In 2000, Healthy People 2010's goal was to decrease the incidence of amputation among patients with diabetes from 4.1 per 1000 (2000) to 1.8 per 1000 (2010).[7,8] A summary of Healthy People 2010 revealed that the rate of lower-extremity amputations in patients with diabetes did in fact decline by 47% from 1997–1999 to 2005–2007. This finding was reflected in an incidence rate reduction from 6.6 per 1000 in 1997 to 3.5 per 1000 population in 2005 (age adjusted).[7] Additionally, females had a lower rate (2.2 per 1000 population [age adjusted]) of lower-extremity amputations than males (4.8 per 1000) in 2005 to 2007.[7] Because of the decline in the rate of amputations among patients with diabetes and its positive implications on health policy, this objective is maintained as a goal for Healthy People 2020.[7]

Goldberg and colleagues[8] (2012) evaluated the effect of the Healthy People 2010 initiative in an enhanced sample of all patients with diabetes from the Medicare 5% sample during 1999 to 2006. They found that the amputation rate declined among patients with diabetes. However, the incidence of amputations among patients with diabetes with greater than 3 comorbidities and end-stage renal disease (ESRD) increased from 1999 to 2006 (**Fig. 2**). This finding offers the perspective that perhaps

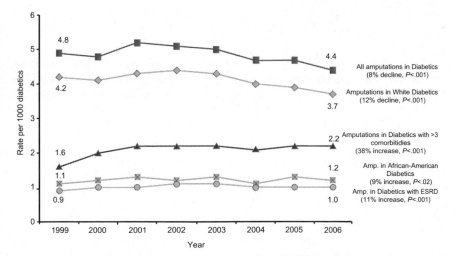

Fig. 2. Temporal trends of amputations in individuals with diabetes by race and comorbidity status. (*From* Goldberg JB, Goodney PP, Cronenwett JL, et al. The effect of risk and race on lower extremity amputations among Medicare diabetic patients. J Vasc Surg 2012;56(6):1665; with permission.)

it is not just a single comorbid condition but rather the combined illness burden from multiple conditions that leads to amputation. Eggers and colleagues[9] (1999) reported from Medicare data that patients with diabetes and ESRD had a 10-fold greater risk of amputation than those with diabetes mellitus without ESRD. This finding suggests that a greater illness burden has serious implications to health care policy beyond the prevention of single diseases.

Within the veteran population, Tseng and colleagues[10] (2011) found that improvements in the early detection and diagnosis of diabetes increased the overall diabetic population that was identified during a time period. This increased denominator serves to lower the rate of lower-extremity amputations. However, Tseng and colleagues[10] further demonstrated with their study conducted within the Veterans Health Administration (VHA) system in New Jersey (2000–2004) that after adjusting for population characteristics and risk factors associated with amputations, there was a persistent decrease in the amputation rates from 7.0 per 1000 to 4.6 per 1000 (reflecting a 34% decrease) among patients with diabetes. Of these amputations, the rates of transfemoral decreased more (49% reduction) than transtibial (19% reduction). One potential contributor to these decreasing rates could be the implementation of a universal program for foot screening within the VHA. In contrast to this study at the VHA, Healthy People 2010 did not note any changes in the percentage of people with diabetes who received annual foot examinations.[7]

In 2009, the hospital costs associated with amputation totaled more than $8.3 billion in the United States.[11] Kurichi and colleagues[12] conducted a study in the VHA to evaluate the factors associated with these costs. Amputations that were associated with systemic sepsis and comorbidities of arrhythmia, chronic blood loss anemia, fluid and electrolyte disorders, and weight loss were associated with both higher total inpatient costs and longer lengths of stay. Amputations caused by certain chronic conditions (osteomyelitis and hypertension) were associated with both lower inpatient costs and shorter lengths of stay. These associations are logical because amputations related to osteomyelitis are often trauma related and occur in younger patients.

PAD

When in its end stage, PAD can lead to lower-extremity amputations.[13] PAD and lower-extremity amputation rates were evaluated among elderly patients using Medicare part A beneficiary data from 2000 to 2008 by Jones and colleagues[14] (2012). They found a decline in the overall annual rate of amputations in patients with PAD from 7258 per 100,000 to 5790 per 100,000 among patients with PAD over that 8-year period. Male sex, black race, diabetes mellitus, and renal disease were all independent predictors of lower-extremity amputation in this PAD population.[14] Geographic variation was also found to play a role in the number of amputations because lower-extremity amputations were more often performed in the East South Central and West South Central regions and less in the mid-Atlantic region when compared with the South Atlantic region.[14]

Limitations remain in the research on peripheral vascular disease and limb loss. Ephraim and colleagues[15] attribute some of these limitations to difficulties identifying people with dysvascular disease by using the *International Classification of Diseases, Ninth Revision* codes. Because of the variations in interpreting these codes, the sample selections vary across studies, making comparisons across them difficult.[15,16]

REAMPUTATION RATES

Reamputation and mortality rates are important to evaluate when considering rates of amputations. In 1980, Ebskov and Josephsen[17] reported from the 1972 Danish Amputation Register that the incidence of ipsilateral reamputation is high in the immediate postoperative period, with 10.4% after 1 month, 16.5% after 3 months, and 18.8% after 6 months. After 4 years, the incidence was 23.1%. However, the contralateral limb's risk of amputation is constantly present, with an incidence of 11.9% within 1 year, 17.8% after 2 years, 27.2% after 3 years, and 44.3% after 4 years.[17] Similarly, Dillingham, Pezzin, and Shore[18] evaluated Medicare beneficiaries' data from the Centers for Medicare and Medicaid Services in 1996 who underwent lower-limb amputations and evaluated the rates of reamputation, mortality, and health care costs within a 12-month period after the initial amputation. They found that 26% required a subsequent amputation procedure. Reamputations were commonly seen among patients with diabetes, and progression occurred most frequently (34.5%) among patients with an initial foot or ankle amputation. Those patients with index amputations at transtibial and transfemoral levels experienced significantly lower rates of reamputations, suggesting that higher levels may provide the highest probability of successful wound healing when compared with either foot or ankle amputations.[18]

TRAUMA

Trauma is the second most common cause of amputations, yet occurs at about one-eighth of the frequency as dysvascular amputations overall. Dillingham, Pezzin, and MacKenzie[19] examined population-based hospital discharge data for Maryland from 1979 through 1993. The incidence of major amputations declined 3.4% annually and 4.8% annually for minor amputations (**Table 2**).[19] Although PAD and diabetes were most commonly associated with lower-limb amputations, upper-limb amputations accounted for the vast majority (68.6%) of all trauma-related amputations.[3] The incidence rates were lower in 1996 relative to 1988, with the exception of (through-knee, pelvic, wrist, transradial, and shoulder amputations).[3] The most notable reduction was the incidence of hand amputations. The researchers attributed this downward trend to potential changes in aggressiveness of both reconstructive (limb salvage) surgery and reimplantation of severed digits.[3] This decline could also be attributed to the improvements in occupational safety standards and the reduction in the proportion of the workforce operating heavy machinery and working in factories. The decline in rates of minor amputations could be partially caused by the increasing use of outpatient care for such severed digits such that these cases are not represented in hospital discharge data.[3]

Gender and race play a role in traumatic amputations.[19–21] Males were at a significantly higher risk double that of trauma-related amputations in females.[19–21] Ebskov,

Table 2			
Traumatic amputation (rates per 100,000 population)			
		Incidence 1979	Incidence 1993
Major amputations	992	1.88	1.07 (38% decline)
Minor amputation	5077	10.8	4.7 (48% decline)
Total	6069	12.7	5.8

From Dillingham TR, Pezzin LE, MacKenzie EJ. Incidence, acute care length of stay, and discharge to rehabilitation of traumatic amputee patients: an epidemiologic study. Arch Phys Med Rehabil 1998;79:281; with permission.

Schroeder, and Holstein[20] reported 2 peaks in the age distribution for men with traumatic amputations from 20 to 29 years of age and 70 to 79 years of age and among women aged 70 to 79 years. The younger age group could be attributed to occupational and automobile accidents and the later peak could be attributed to falls.[19,20] Racial differences were again noted between blacks and nonblacks.[19,20] Dillingham, Pezzin, and MacKenzie[6] reported that blacks older than 35 years were at a higher risk for trauma-related amputations.

Another population that has suffered from traumatic amputations is the postwar-returning veterans. Often the veterans are returning with polytrauma and, thus, necessitating comprehensive care. An estimated 6000 amputations occurred during the Vietnam War.[22] As of December 2012, the Congressional Research Service reports the number of wounded soldiers from Operation Iraqi Freedom (OIF) and Operation Enduring Freedom (OEF) was 18,230; among these injured soldiers, there were 1715 amputations.[23] Pasquina and colleagues[24] reported that 21% of these veterans had upper-limb amputations, and more than 23% lost more than one limb. Most of these service members sustained multiple injuries. Fully 50% of these soldiers with amputations had a documented traumatic brain injury or a vision or hearing deficit. In addition, these amputees suffered from complex fractures, soft tissue wounds, paralysis from peripheral nerve injuries, or spinal cord injuries. There was a high rate of mental health problems, further compounding their recovery and rehabilitation programs.[24] A survey conducted among veterans from OIF/OEF and Vietnam by Reiber and colleagues[25] in 2010 revealed that the veterans from both conflicts experienced limb loss at similar locations, with the most common being transtibial, transfemoral, and transradial. There was, however, a slight increase in transradial and partial foot amputations found in the veterans from the OIF/OEF conflict.

CANCER

Limb loss caused by cancer in the United States is rare compared with dysvascular causes, occurring at less than one-one hundredth the rate of dysvascular amputations. In the United States, primary malignant bone tumors are 6% of all cancers in children younger than 20 years.[26] Osteosarcoma and Ewing sarcoma are the 2 predominant bone malignancies that affect the long bones and central axis.[26] Dillingham, Pezzin, and MacKenzie[3] found that most cancer-related amputations were in the lower extremity, with transfemoral and transtibial amputations accounting for one-third, with no differences in race or gender noted. The decline in the rates of amputation caused by malignancies of the limbs could be caused by advancements in early detection and management of malignancies allowing for surgeons to perform more limb salvage techniques as an alternative to amputations.[26]

CONGENITAL DEFICIENCY

Congenital limb deficiency may be caused by genetic variation, exposure to an environmental teratogen, or gene-environment interactions.[15,16] Birth prevalence rates ranged from 3.5 per 10,000 births (including pregnancy terminations) to 7.1 per 10,000 births.[15,16] The birth prevalence of limb deficiency in children with major congenital anomalies was 12.9 per 10,000 births.[27] Analysis of the HCUP data by Dillingham, Pezzin, and MacKenzie[3] revealed that the incidence of congenital deficiencies accounted for 0.8% of all limb loss–related discharges, which remained stable over the 10-year period.[3] Upper-limb defects occurred more commonly than lower-limb defects.[15] Of these defects, longitudinal hand reductions were most frequent, accounting for 46.4% of the upper-limb anomalies; longitudinal toe reduction was the most common among newborns.[15] There were similar of rates across different countries, with the rate of congenital limb deficiencies falling within 2 to 7 per 10,000 live births.[15]

SUMMARY

Literature from the last 2 decades demonstrates that the rate of amputations among dysvascular patients was 8 times greater than those with trauma-related amputations. However, recent studies have shown a reduction of the rates in subsets of those with diabetes and PAD, which may be attributed to the early detection of conditions and preventive programs. Additionally, the role of a combined illness burden may have a stronger impact on the risk of amputation compared with single disease processes. Being cognizant of the new trends in rates of amputations and their implications will play an integral role in optimizing coordinated health care.

REFERENCES

1. Ziegler-Graham K, MacKenzie EJ, Ephraim PL, et al. Estimating the prevalence of limb loss in the United States: 2005 to 2050. Arch Phys Med Rehabil 2008;89(3): 422–9.
2. Tseng CL, Helmer D, Rajan M, et al. Evaluation of regional variation in total, major, and minor amputation rates in a national health-care system. Int J Qual Health Care 2007;19(6):368–76.
3. Dillingham TR, Pezzin LE, MacKenzie EJ. Limb amputation and limb deficiency: epidemiology and recent trends in the United States. South Med J 2002;95(8): 875–83.
4. National diabetes fact sheet 2011. Available at: http://www.cdc.gov/diabetes/ pubs/pdf/ndfs_2011.pdf. Accessed June 3, 2013.
5. Carmona GA, Hoffmeyer P, Hermann FR, et al. Major lower limb amputations in the elderly observed over ten years: the role of diabetes and peripheral arterial disease. Diabetes Meta 2005;31(5):449–54.
6. Dillingham TR, Pezzin LE, MacKenzie E. Racial differences in the incidence of limb loss secondary to peripheral vascular disease: a population-based study. Arch Phys Med Rehabil 2002;83:1252–7.
7. CDC – Healthy people 2010. Final review. Available at: http://www.cdc.gov/nchs/ healthy_people/hp2010/hp2010_final_review.htm. Accessed May 15, 2013.
8. Goldberg JB, Goodney PP, Cronenwett JL, et al. The effect of risk and race on lower extremity amputations among Medicare diabetic patients. J Vasc Surg 2012;56(6):1663–8.
9. Eggers PW, Ghodes D, Pugh J. Non-traumatic lower extremity amputation in the end stage renal disease Medicare population. Kidney Int 1999;56:1524–33.
10. Tseng CL, Rajan M, Miller DR, et al. Trends in initial lower extremity amputation rates among Veterans Health Administration health care systems users from 2000–2004. Diabetes Care 2011;34(5):1157–63.
11. Amputee coalition: limb loss resource center. Limb loss statistics. 2013. Available at: http://www.amputee-coalition.org/limb-loss-resource-center/resources-by-topic/limb-loss-statistics/limb-loss-statistics/index.html. Accessed May 30, 2013.
12. Kurichi JE, Vogel WB, Kwong PL, et al. Factors associated with total inpatient costs and length of stay during surgical hospitalization among veterans who underwent lower extremity amputation. Am J Phys Med Rehabil 2013;92(3): 203–11.

13. Norgren L, Hiatt WR, Dormandy JA, et al. Inter-society consensus for the management of peripheral arterial disease (TASC II). J Vasc Surg 2007; 45(Suppl S):S5–67.

14. Jones WS, Patel MR, Dai D, et al. Temporal trends and geographic variation of lower-extremity amputation in patients with peripheral artery disease: results from U.S. Medicare 2000-2008. J Am Coll Cardiol 2012;60(21):2230–6.

15. Ephraim PL, Dillingham TR, Sector M, et al. Epidemiology of limb loss and congenital limb deficiency: a review of the literature. Arch Phys Med Rehabil 2003;84(5):747–61.

16. Kurichi J, Stineman M, Kwong PL, et al. Assessing and using comorbidity measures in elderly veterans with lower extremity amputations. Gerontology 2007; 53:255–9.

17. Ebskov B, Josephsen P. Incidence of reamputation and death after gangrene of the lower extremity. Prosthet Orthot Int 1980;4(2):77–80.

18. Dillingham TR, Pezzin LE, Shore AD. Reamputation, mortality, and health care costs among persons with dysvascular lower-limb amputations. Arch Phys Med Rehabil 2005;86(3):480–6.

19. Dillingham TR, Pezzin LE, MacKenzie EJ. Incidence, acute care length of stay, and discharge to rehabilitation of traumatic amputee patients: an epidemiologic study. Arch Phys Med Rehabil 1998;79:279–87.

20. Ebskov LB, Schroeder TV, Holstein PE. Epidemiology of leg amputations: the influence of vascular surgery. Br J Surg 1994;81(11):1600–3.

21. Pohjolainen T, Alaranta H. Lower limb amputations in Southern Finland 1984–1985. Prosthet Orthot Int 1988;12:9–18.

22. Traumatic amputations and prosthetics. Veteran's health initiative. 2002. Available at: http://www.publichealth.va.gov/docs/vhi/traumatic_amputation.pdf. Accessed June 18, 2013.

23. Fischer H. Congressional research service report. 2013. Available at: http://www.fas.org/sgp/crs/natsec/RS22452.pdf. Accessed May 18, 2013.

24. Pasquina PF, Scoville CR, Belnap B et al. Introduction: developing a combat system of care for the combat amputee. Available at: https://ke.army.mil/bordeninstitute/published_volumes/amputee/CCAchapter01.pdf. Accessed May 10, 2013.

25. Reiber GE, McFarland LV, Hubbard S, et al. Service members and veterans with major traumatic limb loss from Vietnam War and OIF/OEF conflicts: survey methods, participants, and summary findings. J Rehabil Res Dev 2010;47: 275–98.

26. Nagarajan R, Neglia JP, Clohisty DR. Limb salvage and amputation in survivors of pediatric lower extremity bone tumors: what are the long-term implications? J Clin Oncol 2002;22:4493–501.

27. Rosano A, Botto L, Onlye R, et al. Limb defects associated with major congenital anomalies: clinical and epidemiological study from the international clearinghouse for birth defects monitoring systems. Am J Med Genet 2000;93:110–6.

Impact of Limb Loss in the United States

Terrence Patrick Sheehan, MD[a,b,]*, George C. Gondo, MA[b]

KEYWORDS

- Prosthetics • Limb loss • Amputees • US health care system

KEY POINTS

- The amputee gets lost in the American health care system because of fragmentation across the continuum, especially those that are diabetic related but includes those that are trauma related.
- The journey of the diabetic patient with limb loss through the US health care system is even more precarious than that of the traumatic amputee.
- Interventions to address these secondary conditions and improve the health and outcomes of persons with disability have focused on standard medical treatments, such as medication or physical rehabilitation therapies, often to the exclusion of psychosocial interventions.
- Each member of the amputee rehabilitation team, if trained well, plays a specific and important role in the care and recovery of the person with limb loss.

The amputation of a limb represents a rare disease that has significant burden on the US health care system. Amputation rates in the total population, including individuals without diabetes, those with peripheral arterial disease (PAD) alone, and those that are cancer related, are not known. But it is startling to understand that estimates of 300 to more than 500 amputations occur in the United States every day. No active surveillance efforts, such as registry, currently exist. In this respect, those with limb loss in America have been forgotten in the health care system. A registry would give a clear picture of the landscape of limb loss in America and provide data to support research and help establish evidence-based interventions for patients with limb loss. To form and maintain a registry takes an act of Congress with a line item approved by the US congressional appropriations committee. From the respected research that has been done, it is estimated that nearly 2 million persons are living with limb loss in the United States.[1] It is projected that the number of people living with the loss of a limb will more than double by 2050.[1] According to recent data, more than 147,000

a Adventist Rehabilitation Hospital of Maryland, 9909 Medical Center Drive, Rockville, MD 20850, USA; b Amputee Coalition of America, 9303 Center Street, Suite 100, Manassas, VA 20110, USA
* Corresponding author. Amputee Coalition of America, 9303 Center Street, Suite 100, Manassas, VA 20110.
E-mail address: TSheehan@ahm.com

Phys Med Rehabil Clin N Am 25 (2014) 9–28
http://dx.doi.org/10.1016/j.pmr.2013.09.007
1047-9651/14/$ – see front matter © 2014 Elsevier Inc. All rights reserved.

amputation procedures were performed in the United States in 2010.[2] Of these procedures, more than 57,000 or nearly 40% were performed on patients with a principal diagnosis of diabetes.[2] The costs associated with limb loss in terms of health care expenditures and on the burden of disease on those who have a limb amputated are staggering. Annually, the immediate health care costs associated with the amputation of a limb, not including prosthetic or rehabilitation costs, total nearly than $8 billion.[2] When the costs of prosthetic care, rehabilitation, and other health care costs are accounted for, the economic costs associated with amputation are significantly higher. It is estimated that the 5-year health care costs associated with limb loss are more than $500,000 per person, nearly double the lifetime health care costs of an average person.[3,4] In addition, the 5-year prosthetic costs for a person with limb loss are estimated to be as high as $450,000.[5] The health care costs associated with limb loss are further compounded by the disease burden on those who have a limb amputation.

People with limb loss must often manage multiple chronic health conditions, face an elevated risk for developing even more chronic health conditions, and experience mortality rates higher than many common chronic diseases. The amputation of a limb is frequently an outcome of an existing chronic condition (eg, diabetes or vascular disease). Additionally, having limb loss itself is associated with many chronic conditions. People who have a limb amputated are at an increased risk of cardiovascular disease,[6] obesity,[7] joint and bone issues,[8] and experience high rates of depression and emotional distress.[9] People with limb loss also experience 5-year mortality rates higher than many cancers. Studies estimate the 5-year mortality rate of people with limb loss to be between 50% and 74%.[10] For patients who are 65 years or older and have a limb amputation due to vascular disease, the 1-year mortality rate is estimated to be 36%. This mortality rate increases with the increasing level of amputation. Those who lose a limb due to complications related to diabetes are also predicted to suffer subsequent amputation to either the ipsilateral or contralateral limb within the years following the initial amputation.[11] Their only hope is focused prevention strategy.

TRAUMATIC LIMB LOSS

Patients with an amputation get lost in the American health care system because of fragmentation across the continuum, including those who lost a limb due to trauma. Trauma is the second leading cause of amputation in the United States. About 30,000 traumatic amputations occur in this country every year. Four of every 5 traumatic amputation victims are male, and most of them are between the ages of 15 and 30. Based on the National Trauma Databank version 5 from 2000 to 2004, there were 8910 patients who had an amputation (1.0% of all trauma patients). Of these, 76.9% had digit and 23.1% had limb amputation. Of those with limb amputation, 92.7% had a single limb amputation. Lower extremity amputations (LEA) were more frequent than upper extremity amputation (UEA) among patients in the single limb amputation group (58.9% vs 41.1%). The mechanism of injury was blunt trauma in 83%; most commonly after motor vehicle collisions (51.0%), followed by machinery accidents (19.4%). Motor vehicle collision occupants had more UEA (54.5% vs 45.5%), whereas motorcyclists (86.2% vs 13.8%) and pedestrians (91.9% vs 8.1%) had more LEA. Patients with LEA were more likely to require discharge to a "skilled nursing facility"; whereas those with UEA were more likely to be discharged home.[12] Traumatic limb amputation is not uncommon after trauma in the civilian population and is associated with significant morbidity. The person who experiences a traumatic limb amputation is initially dependent on the surgical trauma team with regard to medical knowledge, skill, and ability to programmatically access a full complement of resources to care for this individual with limb loss. The initial events are centered on sustaining life, then on complex decisions of possible limb salvage and residual limb preservation. This phase can last less than 24 hours or years depending on circumstances and health care team guidance.

The numbers of those with major traumatic limb loss are relatively small, especially when considering that they are spread throughout the United States. This impacts the trauma team's experience regarding decisions of limb preservation as well as technical skill for performing major limb amputation. The approach and outcomes are variable in the United States. Using the recommended standardized surgical techniques for closure and neuroma prevention, when possible, is paramount to meet the goal of functional restoration. As the acute trauma team moves from viewing the amputation as "a therapeutic failure" to "the best therapeutic option," planning for functional restoration comes more clearly into view.

The patients journey in the US health care system after the amputation is one even more variable than the initial immediate trauma phase. The Emergency Medical System directs those at risk to "trauma centers," where it is implied that standardized programs and a full cadre of specialists are ready to care for the trauma victim. The expectation is that after the "usual trauma care" the person with limb loss will be embraced by a comprehensive and cohesive team of rehabilitation professionals with extensive experience. Their experience is evident through a defined program spanning from the time of limb loss through lifetime care, with links to the larger health care system. This is often not the case, even when the person is initially admitted to one of the most sophisticated health care systems in one of the most affluent cities in the United States. It would follow that if it is not happening in one of the "Top Hospitals" it is again unlikely that such a program is "usual care" in the regional trauma centers throughout these United States. The person with limb loss and their supports string together the health care providers who assist them with obtaining therapy services, a prosthesis, progressive healing, and pain management. Significant time is lost without a navigator and a defined amputee specialty care team.

There are few Amputee Specialty Programs in the United States, as they are not "usual care," except in the Department of Veterans Affairs (VA) system. The journey of functional restoration and maximizing quality outcomes for the person with traumatic limb loss is usually in the hands of the person with limb loss and the soloed individual health care providers and prosthetists that he or she encounters. Programmatic components that have been found to be significantly beneficial for the person with limb loss,[13] such as ones that address adjustment, depression, pain, and valuable peer support, do not exist in the "usual care" experience in the United States. The outcomes for functional restoration after traumatic amputation are at risk and variable. The Department of Defense hospitals and the VA hospitals have produced successful programs, benchmarks, and outcomes that need to be translated into "usual care" in our civilian health care system.

NONTRAUMATIC LIMB LOSS
Peripheral Arterial Disease

Lower-extremity PAD is a serious disease that affects approximately 8 to 12 million Americans. Prevalence increases dramatically with age and disproportionately affects African-Americans.[14] The hardened arteries found in people with PAD may be the first sign that a person has a systemic process of hardened and narrowed arteries, supplying critical organs such as the heart and the brain, threatening life not just limb. As a result, people with PAD who are at risk for limb loss are also at high risk for having a heart attack or a stroke. Conversely, but not as frequently recognized, 40% of patients with coronary artery disease (CAD) have PAD.[15]

There is significant overlap, as the evidenced-based treatment of one treats the other. The signs and symptoms of PAD may not arise until later in life. For many, the outward indications will not appear until the artery has narrowed by 60% or more. One in 3 people age 70 or older has PAD. The disease prevalence increases with age and approximately 20% of Americans age 65 and older have PAD. As the population ages, the prevalence could reach up to 16 million in those older than age 65. Of all people with PAD, 2% will progress to major amputation.[16] One method the body uses to adapt to the narrowed arteries is the development of smaller peripheral arteries that allow blood flow around the narrowed area. This process is known as collateral circulation and may help explain why many can have PAD without feeling any symptoms. When a piece of cholesterol, calcium, or blood clot abruptly breaks from the lining of the artery or a narrowed artery blocks off completely, blood flow will be totally obstructed and the organ supplied by that artery will suffer damage. The organs in PAD most commonly affected and researched are the legs. The most advanced stages of PAD can lead to critical limb ischemia (CLI). The pain caused by CLI can wake up an individual at night. This pain, also called "rest pain," can be relieved temporarily by hanging the leg over the bed or getting up to walk around. The legs and feet have such severe blockage that they do not receive the oxygen-rich blood required for basic mobility and cannot repair openings in the skin. This often progresses to a very painful pivotal ischemic episode resulting in amputation. A recent study indicates that early revascularization may prevent this progression.[17] Revascularization was associated with a 40% reduction in amputation rates in patients with PAD, according to research that evaluated 1906 procedures over 2 decades. The investigators found that as use of revascularization to improve circulation rose, the amputation rate dropped. The study covered 1990 to 2009.

The prevalence of PAD is 20% higher in the diabetic population.[15] People with diabetic-related amputation have a significant degree of PAD but there is a distinct group of amputees who have PAD alone. Some studies have found that 1 of 3 people older than 50 with diabetes has PAD, and PAD is even more common in African American and Hispanic patients who have diabetes. People who have both diseases are much more likely to have a heart attack or stroke than those who have PAD alone. Because many people with diabetes do not have feeling in their feet or legs due to nerve disease, they may have PAD but cannot feel any symptoms. Ankle brachial index is a simple, sensitive, and specific test that is essential for primary health care providers to use as a screen. Guidelines released by leading vascular organizations recommend that people older than 50 with diabetes are tested for PAD. Testing is also recommended for people younger than 50 with diabetes and with other risk factors, such as smoking, high blood pressure, or cholesterol problems. PAD warning signs, which include fatigue and tiredness or pain in your feet, legs, thighs, or buttocks that always happens when you walk but that goes away when you rest, cannot be ignored. Unfortunately, most people with PAD do not have any symptoms until the disease is significantly advanced.

Diabetes

Diabetes is a leading cause of nontraumatic lower extremity amputations (NLEAs). Rates of NLEAs serve as an important gauge of the effectiveness of efforts to reduce diabetes complications because they are associated with numerous modifiable risk factors, including high blood pressure, high lipid and glycemic levels, and screening and care for high-risk feet.[18] The number of US residents with diagnosed diabetes increased dramatically from 5.4 million in 1988 to 26.0 million in 2012, or 8% of the population. The estimated number of diabetes-related NLEAs has been reported to be approximately 200 a day in the United States. One recent study found that the rate of amputation may be declining among Americans with diabetes.[19]

Rates of foot and leg amputations among Americans with diabetes may vary widely according to where they live. In a recent study, researchers found that in some parts of the country the rate can be almost double the national average, at least among older Americans.[20] The investigators reported that in 2008, certain pockets of Arkansas, Louisiana, Mississippi, Oklahoma, and Texas had the highest rates of diabetes-related amputation among Medicare beneficiaries at approximately 7.5 per 1000. That compared with a national rate of 4.5 per 1000 in the same year. Certain locations, such as portions of Arizona, Florida, Michigan, and New Mexico, had particularly low rates. There, older adults with diabetes had amputations at a rate of 2.4 to 3.5 per 1000.

In very basic terms, amputation is a complication of diabetes because the disease often causes nerve damage over time. The architecture of the foot changes and thus the standard contoured shoe becomes an ill-fitting shoe and a source of injury to the foot. When people lose sensation in their feet and legs, they may not notice an abrasion, blister, or sore. Most people without normal pain sensation are less likely to notice, become alarmed, and get help until the injury becomes infected. Those wounds can be difficult to heal because diabetes often causes poor blood circulation to the distal lower limbs. A large number persons with diabetic-related limb loss do not seek attention for their foot until presenting to the emergency department with extensive infection and/or irreversible ischemia. Infection spreads into the deep tissues, often quickly, and in many cases amputation of part of the foot or leg is necessary to prevent a dangerous, systemic infection.

It is unusual to find a diabetic patient with limb loss who understood before the amputation that he or she was at significant risk for limb loss because of diabetes. The usual response is that "I had no idea this could happen," even though it is known that limb amputation rate is 8 times higher among people with diabetes than the nondiabetic population.[19] This is a failure of understanding and information transfer by our health care professionals to those who are at risk: the patients they serve.

Obesity

Limb loss and "the obesity paradox"

Two-thirds of US adults are overweight or obese.[21] If obesity rates continue on their current trajectories, by 2030, 13 states could have adult obesity rates higher than 60%, 39 states could have rates higher than 50%, and all 50 states could have rates higher than 44%. The number of obese adults, along with related disease rates and health care costs, are on course to increase dramatically in every state in the country over the next 20 years, according to *F as in Fat: How Obesity Threatens America's Future 2012*.[22] This report suggests that states could prevent obesity-related diseases and dramatically reduce health care costs if they reduced the average body mass index (BMI) of their residents by just 5% by 2030.

Obesity is a precursor to adult-onset diabetes. It has been well established that obesity promotes insulin resistance through the inappropriate inactivation of a gluconeogenesis, where the liver creates glucose for fuel and which ordinarily occurs only in times of fasting. One would predict higher rates of NLEA, given this significant link and epidemic of those with obesity and related diabetes. Paradoxically, a recent study has shown a higher BMI is associated with lower 5-year NLEA risk among nonelderly diabetic men. Individuals with BMI (morbidly obese) of 40.0 kg/m^2 or higher are almost half as likely to have any or major NLEA at the 5-year follow-up than those with BMI (overweight) of 25.0 to 29.9 kg/m^2. These results run counter to an extensive body of literature that suggests obesity is associated with adverse health outcomes in the general population as well as among diabetic patients.

It needs to be highlighted that this nonelderly population is in contrast to the elderly diabetic population who experience most of the limb loss in the United States. It is unclear if the morbidly obese survive to these older ages, as according to the National Obesity Observatory, life expectancy is reduced 10 years for those with a BMI higher than 40 kg/m^2. This paradox is also interesting when considering the finding that showed a significant J-shaped association between BMI and foot ulceration. Those with BMI higher than 40 kg/m^2 were found to be twice more likely to develop foot ulceration during a 5-year follow-up than overweight individuals.[23] Because foot ulcers are the single most important risk for NLEA, results that showed decreasing NLEA risk with increasing BMI are unexpected. The reason for the paradox is yet to be explained; possibly, severely obese individuals experience more foot ulceration as well as better wound healing than individuals with lower BMI.

Weight gain after limb loss

Those with limb loss have been found to be at particular risk of developing an increase in body fat after amputation along with the associated obesity-related diseases. Given the limb loss and change in body mass there is no current accurate BMI guide that defines one across the spectrum as underweight through morbidly obese. Despite this, a study of NLEA among participants in the National Health and Nutrition Examination Survey (NHANES) Epidemiologic Follow-up Study found that people with lower extremity amputation had a higher baseline BMI than those without a lower extremity amputation.[24] The increases in body fat have been linked directly with higher amputation level. The frequency of obesity increased with the level of amputation. For example, obesity rates in those with unilateral transtibial amputation equaled 37.9%; in those with transfemoral amputation, 48.0%; and in subjects with bilateral transfemoral or transfemoral plus transtibial amputation, 64.2%. Obesity progressed early during the first year after amputation.[7] BMI failed to correlate with functional outcome and, specifically, obesity did not predict a poorer prognosis.[25]

In a comprehensive rehabilitation program it is important to start education and counseling regarding nutrition, exercise, and the threat of obesity. Creating understanding of the significant threat of obesity after limb loss allows the patient with limb loss to make better choices. It also allows the rehabilitation team to set goals not just around mobility but about weight control and cardiovascular health. In a comprehensive amputee specialty program in which lifetime follow-up is possible, monitoring weight gain and providing strategies for control are integral interventions. Weight gain of as little as 10 pounds can change the customized fit of the socket causing skin irritation and gait dysfunction.

HEALTH DISPARITY

In the United States there is a significant health disparities exist within the limb loss community, as 42% of those with limb loss are identified as belonging to a racial or ethnic minority group (LLTF). Even though access to care has improved remarkably for racial minorities over the past 2 decades, it is known that minorities are disproportionately affected by multiple barriers to care: grounded in financial, language, cultural, logistical, organizational, institutional, and systemic differences. Providing adequate access to care may not be sufficient to eliminate ethnic disparities in health. In the Health Disparities and Inequities Report of 2011 by the Centers for Disease Control and Prevention (CDC), minority groups were overrepresented in every diagnostic category monitored except suicide and drug-induced death, where whites prevailed.[26] Minorities have been noted to participate to a greater extent in adverse health risk behaviors, demonstrate decreased compliance with prescribed medical treatment, and have concerns about their ability to trust medical providers.[27] African-American and Hispanic individuals were less likely to use most preventive services when compared with non-Hispanic white individuals.[28]

African American Individuals

Higher amputation rates among black patients may be the result of less aggressive limb salvage care. Black patients with PAD undergo amputation at 2 to 4 times the rate of white patients.[29] Black and Hispanic patients with PAD and diabetes experience a greater incidence and odds of amputation when compared with non-Hispanic white patients. In addition, the literature also supports a greater severity of amputation as expressed by higher amputation levels among minorities compared with non-Hispanic white patients. Black female patients have been reported to have greater than 7 times the rate of amputation than white women. Several studies have reported minority patients are much less likely to receive preventive vascular screenings and procedures.[30] Black patients are much less likely than white patients to undergo attempts at limb salvage before amputation. Elderly black amputees were significantly less likely than white amputees to have undergone 1, 2, 3, or more revascularizations before amputation.

Many studies have evaluated what happens to black and white patients who presented to a hospital with limb ischemia. In general, these studies have shown that black patients more frequently undergo amputation, and white patients more frequently undergo revascularization.[31,32] Whether this disparity can be attributable to race-related differences in severity of arterial disease, patient preferences, or physician decision making is unclear. Reasons for this disparity are likely to include differences in insurance coverage, socioeconomic status, comorbid conditions, or pattern or severity of disease at presentation, but studies have not been able to eliminate a persistent difference in amputation rates due to race.[33] It is unknown if a biologic difference in the pattern or progression of arterial disease among black compared with white patients exists that may preclude revascularization as a viable means of preventing or delaying amputation. Data suggest that black patients do not present later with more advanced disease than white patients as an explanation of this disparity. It is interesting that toe amputation is the single procedure for which black and white patients saw similar rates before major lower extremity amputation, which suggests a true racial disparity with regard to attempts at limb salvage before major amputation in the black population.[30] Shamefully, with this overwhelming amount of data and evidence there is no concerted, focused program in the United States addressing limb loss among minority groups; particularly in the African American subgroup. This is another example of the person at risk for limb loss or with limb loss being forgotten in our fragmented health care system.

Native Americans

Diabetes is the fourth leading cause of death among American Indians and Alaska Natives, and mortality due to diabetes among American Indians and Alaska Natives is 4 times higher than that of the US general population.[34] Heart disease, the leading cause of American Indian and Alaska Native mortality, appears to be more often fatal among American Indians than in other populations. The morbidity burden among the American Indian with diabetes exceeded that of other US adults with diabetes by 50%.

American Indian adults with diabetes were significantly more likely to have renal failure, lower-extremity amputations, and neuropathy than were other US adults with diabetes. The rate for amputations among American Indian adults was greater than 10 times that of other US adults.[35] The Strong Heart Study is a study of cardiovascular disease and its risk factors in 13 American Indian communities. Data on the presence or absence of amputations were collected at each of 3 serial examinations (1989–1992, 1993–1995, and 1997–1999) by direct examination of the lower extremity. Of the 1974 individuals with diabetes and without NLEA at baseline, 87 (4.4%) experienced an LEA during 8 years of follow-up. Amputation of toes was most common, followed by transtibial and transfemoral amputations. Odds of LEA were higher among individuals with unfavorable combinations of risk factors, such as high ankle-brachial index (1.40), longer duration of diabetes, less than a high school education, and elevated HbA(1c). The adjusted risk of LEA in men was twice that of women. For the Native American patients there has been educational programmatic outreach by the CDC through the Amputee Coalition. This can be a model used for other minority groups at risk.

The Importance of Focused Education

The importance of education in reducing risk of LEA was shown in a previous study of black and white Americans in the NHANES Epidemiologic Follow-up Study. This study showed that although there were substantially higher age-adjusted rates of lower extremity amputation in African-Americans, compared with white Americans, this excess risk was eliminated when the presence of a high school education was considered, along with age, diabetes, smoking, and hypertension. Of particular interest in this report and the Strong Heart Study is the nearly identical adjusted risk estimates associated with having a high school education: in the NHANES Follow-up Study, the adjusted risk estimate for LEA associated with having completed high school was 0.47, and the corresponding risk estimate in the Strong Heart Study was 0.46. Thus, in African-American and American Indian populations, completing high school reduces the risk of LEA by greater than 50%.[24] Understanding the importance of education and specifically the risk level for those who have not completed a high school level of education allows public health measures to be targeted and efficient. Finally, the higher risk in American Indian males compared with females is interesting and may be related to more severe peripheral neuropathy. For example it is known that there is less peripheral neuropathy and lower rates of NLEA in diabetic South Asians compared to Europeans. It is also possible that men experience more minor trauma to the foot that ultimately results in NLEA. Both of which stress the importance of identifying the neuropathy early in those at risk and educating those at higher risk for limb loss about importance of monitoring their feet at all times.

PREVENTABLE LIMB LOSS

The journey of the patient with diabetes with limb loss through the US health care system is even more precarious than that of the traumatic amputee. Although not all cases of limb loss are preventable, the leading cause of amputation, complications from diabetes and peripheral vascular disease, can often be prevented through patient education, disease management, and regular foot screening. Preventable limb loss is especially important to racial and ethnic minority groups, where the amputation rate is up to 10 times that of white Americans. Among people with diabetes and peripheral vascular disease, early intervention and increased patient education have been associated with reducing the incidence of amputation. Recent research showing 67%

decline in the rate of lower limb amputation from diabetes-related complications since 1996 demonstrates the potential efficacy of prevention efforts.[19] Yet the number of diabetes-related complications remains high and the prevalence of diabetes and chronic kidney disease has grown tremendously. In 2009, there were an estimated 68,000 diabetes-related major limb amputations performed in the United States, a 23% increase since 1988.[36] The CDC estimated that more than 20 million Americans had been diagnosed with diabetes in 2010, four times the number of Americans diagnosed with diabetes in 1980.[36] In 2010, nearly 70,000 Americans died due to diabetes, making it the seventh leading cause of death in the United States.[37] Having diabetes is associated with a 55% increase in mortality in people who have a lower-limb amputation.[11]

Early intervention for coronary artery disease and cerebral vascular disease are integral parts of primary care in the US yet this does not exist for PAD, despite epidemics in diabetes and obesity. Patients understand the importance of diabetic foot care better when it is demonstrated by a provider who examines the feet carefully at least annually, and asks about foot problems at every visit.[38] This is not "usual care" in our primary care offices. Of the many that do seek attention for issues related to their feet, it is usually to a single provider, such as a primary care specialist or a podiatrist. It is not "usual care" to send someone at risk for limb loss to a specialized team who collaboratively focus on limb preservation. All too often the person new to limb loss states that he or she had "no idea I was at risk for losing my leg."

Our civilian health care system does not reimburse for care centered on protecting someone who is at significant risk for limb loss. For example, a person found to have a history of diabetes, as well as any and all of the following: hypertension, >100 cigarette lifetime smoking history, sensory-motor peripheral neuropathy, and abnormal (high or low) ankle brachial index (ABI) is at risk for developing ulceration, ischemia, and limb loss. When this is recognized by the primary care physician or specialist there is no reimbursement for the coordination of preventive measures inclusive of vascular evaluation, podiatry intervention, and pedorthotist intervention. There is poor understanding of the impact of simple measures such as the fact that in our Medicare system if you are diabetic you are covered annually for protective footwear; if you have PAD alone, there is no coverage for protective footwear.

Wound care centers have become common in US community hospitals. At wound care centers there is often access to all services and specialists needed for limb loss prevention. Wound centers remain just "wound care" centers as opposed to "limb preservation and wound care centers" because they are reimbursed to take care of a wound. If there is no wound present, there is no reimbursement mechanism to support sending someone to this team. Specifically preventing the precursor to amputation, the callous, the skin irritation, and the ulcer, is dependent on the intervention of the health provider who understands the risk, seeks to intervene early with identifying correctable PAD, facilitating comprehensive preventive education and implementing proven protective measures. A person at risk could not be referred in to the wound center for care navigation, evaluation, and comprehensive following to prevent any opening of the skin of the foot.

It is often too late once the skin is open. It is the callous and ulcer that is the precursor to the infected ischemic foot. It is estimated that 85% of diabetes-related amputations are preceded by a foot ulcer.[39]

We need our wound care centers to evolve into limb preservation centers, with reimbursed navigators and educators. It has been demonstrated that a collaborative team-based approach is needed to preserve a limb. This team should consist of a primary care specialist, wound care specialist, infectious disease specialist, vascular disease specialist, and pedorthotist. The emphasis first needs to be on preventing skin open-ing, then on removing barriers to healing, including infection, poor perfusion, and un-controlled systemic diseases, as well as an emphasis on proven care interventions (eg, dressings, hyperbaric treatments). Patient-centered education is critical to fully engage the person being served, as well as for team communication.

Diabetic foot care self-management education activities and programs can improve foot care behaviors and decrease lower limb morbidities.[38] This model has been demonstrated in the VA medical centers, in which risk identification and collaborative care, along with using the system's electronic medical record, resulted in the ampu-tation rate among patients with diabetes decreasing by more than 50%.[10] The VA demonstrated that once a person was identified in the health record with risk factors, accountable prevention strategies were put in place that reduced ulcer formation, as well as the number and severity of amputations. This centered on collaboration be-tween health care professional and following defined protocols. This is not surprising, as it is estimated that as many as 60% of the amputations resulting from diabetes-related complications could have been prevented.[40] Reducing the number of amputa-tions due to dysvascular disease by 10% can reduce the number of people living with limb loss in the United States in 2050 by 225,000.[1]

"USUAL CARE" IN THE UNITED STATES

Unlike the person who is treated at the trauma center by a trauma team, diabetic-related amputations occur in every acute care hospital in the United States and are performed by a variety surgical specialists (general, vascular, orthopedic, and podi-atric) with variable skill level. There is no designated team assembled, like in trauma centers, and thus protocols are not standardized and the "usual care" is not compre-hensive or standardized. There is no standardized "limb attack" protocol as there is when heart and brain tissue is in jeopardy.

The ultimate outcome for the person who has just lost his or her limb is often depen-dent on the initial interventions. This includes the surgical technique used and, during the acute hospitalization, connections made with the rehabilitation team. If the skill level is marginal and the collaborative care model nonexistent, the amputee's ultimate functional outcome is at risk. As most, 75%, of these persons with new limb loss are older than 65, the resources and settings for postacute care provided are also vari-able. They are dependent on the acute care team having a vision of the potential after limb loss, particularly for an older population. They are dependent on the knowledge base of the acute care team to direct the person with limb loss to the Amputee Spe-cialty Team, if available, or at a minimum to the acute rehabilitation program. For those supported with managed insurance, this pivotal referral is then conditional on an educated insurer allowing this critical path for recovery after limb loss. Often the acute care team does not have a vision of what is possible for the person with limb loss, especially the older amputee, and a nursing facility or home are the only discharge plans made. They get basic discharge instructions: "keep your incision clean, come back in 2 weeks, and good luck." In neither of these settings will the amputee find the knowledgeable team of limb loss rehabilitation specialists, inclusive of the pros-thetist and peer advocate, who all have the vision for what can be achieved after limb loss. This process begins before the staples or sutures are out. All too often the amputation is seen as a clinical failure as opposed to the best treatment option, and the grieving acute care team does little to create an optimistic vision for life after limb loss. Because amputations are an infrequent occurrence in each individual acute care hospital, amputees are spread so thin through our health care system that they are a group that belongs to no specific specialty and no formal programmatic pathways have been developed like the ones for stroke and heart attack in the acute care setting. In today's health care system, the most natural lead is the physiatrist who engineers a comprehensive program for lifetime following and team collaboration. The amputee is the patient with unmet needs specific to his or her recent limb loss in the acute care hospital. It is rare today for a woman with an acute mastectomy to not be visited and cared for by a specialized team ready to meet her immediate postacute needs. This is not the case for the person with a new limb amputation in the acute care hospital.

The postacute continuum has seen improvement. In the acute rehabilitation hospital, certified programs in general rehabilitation, spinal cord injury, and brain injury, have been developed and refined for more than 30 years through the Commission on the Accreditation of Rehabilitation Facilities (CARF). In 2007, an international panel developed the first and only standards of care for the rehabilitation of the person with limb loss. These have been developed and maintained by CARF, whose standards are designed from the "patient experience" perspective and evidenced-based medicine. They were designed to be applied anywhere a team approach is developed in the postacute care continuum, emphasizing person-centered collaborative care with continuity and lifetime follow-up. The prevention of secondary limb loss, of course, is a primary goal in the Amputee Specialty program standards. There are now more than 45 accredited programs in the United States with a high concentration in the VA system, as well as some internationally accredited programs. The VA system in collaboration with the Department of Defense leads the United States in the care of those with limb loss, as well as preventing limb loss.

ADJUSTMENT AFTER LIMB LOSS

Attention to adjustment after limb loss begins with intervention before the amputation, when possible. A psychological consultation before amputation is appropriate, because patients who are unprepared and depressed may experience more physical and psychosocial difficulties afterward.[41] Functional outcome can be improved by appropriately addressing the psychosocial factors, because loss of the ability to relate psychologically, vocationally, avocationally, sexually, and socially after amputation may have more impact on quality of life than the loss of the limb itself.[41] The impact of limb loss extends beyond chronic conditions and mortality rates and deeply penetrates the emotional and psychological well-being of patients. Amputation should be regarded as a therapeutic and reconstructive procedure that is designed to restore function and attempt to allow the patient to return to an independent lifestyle.[42] Interesting but not surprising, studies have noted that when patient with posttraumatic limb salvage were candid, they frequently stated that, although their limbs were saved, their lives were ruined by the prolonged and costly attempts at reconstruction.[43] Patients who are at risk for or sustain amputations should be provided with counseling to address adjustment to disability, depression, and posttraumatic stress disorder.[44] Studies on the social and emotional impact of limb loss suggest that nearly 30% of the population with limb loss experience significant depressive symptoms following their amputation.[45] Experiencing psychosocial distress following the amputation of a limb is thought to be associated with increased intensity and bothersome pain.[46]

Ultimate adjustment to amputation and perceived quality of life are influenced by multiple factors, such as patient's age, level of maturity, past experiences, temperament, inner strength, personality traits, coping strategies, social support, comorbidities, site and cause of amputation, length of time since amputation, and comprehensiveness of care.[41] Caring for the adjustment of the person after limb loss needs to be individualized and extend beyond becoming mobile with a prosthetic. Losing a limb has a significant impact on the social lives of patients with limb loss. People with limb loss perceive that they are participating less in recreational activities, are more dissatisfied at work, and are more impaired in community mobility relative to their premorbid status.[41]

If they are part of a coordinated rehabilitation program available across the continuum, reintegration into the community can be initiated early with the supervision of the team members during such activities as organized trips for shopping, recreation reintroduction, and initiating return to work or school as tolerated. Persons who lose a limb perceive barriers in many domains of social life, especially with encountering difficulties returning to work.[47] Many have to change the nature of their occupation or work part-time.

Interventions to address these secondary conditions and improve the health and outcomes of persons with disability have focused on standard medical treatments, such as medication or physical rehabilitation therapies, often to the exclusion of psychosocial interventions. More recently, however, attention has been directed at supplementing these more traditional approaches with individual and group-based "self- management" (SM) programs that are rooted in the principles of cognitive behavioral therapy and use 2 broad approaches: coping skills training and cognitive restructuring techniques. SM programs can improve the outcomes of persons with limb loss beyond the benefits of traditional support groups.[13] This suggests that the structured, skill-based activities of the SM approach are beneficial beyond the potential nonspecific benefits, including modeling, social support, and informal information sharing, which may amass from peer support groups.

Ever since the bombing at the Boston Marathon, there has been much discussion about the long-term ramifications for the victims who lost limbs. Although there are obviously physical obstacles to navigate, there are often as many psychological hurdles. People have to adjust to a new body image and manage their losses, both of the limb and the changes that amputation causes in their lives. This means learning to manage their depression and anxiety. Pain is particularly common among persons with limb loss, with 65% to 75% of amputees reporting phantom limb, residual limb, or back pain 3 or more years after amputation, the intensity of which is linked to depression and poor adjustment. Given the significant high rates of major depression and pain, programmatic SM interventions significantly impact functional outcome, resulting in fewer restrictions in activities and improved quality of life. Because it is rare for one to have knowledge and preparation before limb loss, whether a traumatic injury or not, the person having experienced the loss of a limb may have to deal with posttraumatic stress issues. People are remarkably resilient and will bounce back quicker than believed after such a devastating loss. Part of their recovery clearly hinges on the support system around them, not to mention their own skill set and coping capacity. With that in mind, patients need help to take charge of their own recovery. SM is grounded in the idea that patients can and should take an active role in managing their condition and recovery. Among other things, SM provides knowledge, training in monitoring their activity or pain levels, problem solving, and practice in other skills needed to function. Those skills could include the most basic things, like planning community activities, or the less concrete, such as relaxation techniques.

Social recovery is dependent on the response and adaption of the other people in the life of the amputee. Integrating the family and supports into the rehabilitation and recovery program is paramount in setting the stage for a healthy adaptation after limb loss. This is a multifaceted biologic, physical, social, and emotional recovery, and it often takes place over the course of months and years. Efforts begin during the patient's hospitalization, if not in the acute phase, then in the postacute phase of a comprehensive rehabilitation program. It is fundamental to have access to the complete team, physicians, therapists, pastoral counselor, and rehabilitation psychologists, but an often pivotal meeting with a peer is crucial. The ability to meet with another, "similar" person with limb loss is a powerful connection. This person brings wisdom and vision in addition to the "been there, done that" factor. The Amputee Coalition is the only national nonprofit advocacy group in the United States that represents the more than 2 million people living with limb loss. The Amputee Coalition, having a keen understanding of the importance of this peer level of advocacy, has developed an award-winning national program for formally training peers to be effective supports to those new to limb loss. Recovery and adjustment needs to be holistic, attending to the entire spectrum of needs. The team, including the person served, works together to facilitate recovery and adaption to life with limb loss. The Amputee Coalition has focused on creating resources that help persons with limb loss manage the struggles associated with amputation, in the voice and perspective of the peer. The "Promoting Amputee Life Skills," (PALS) program, is just one of them. It is a structured weekly group course that meets for 10 weeks. It is facilitated by trained peers and entails a group of amputees helping each other cultivate their SM skills and achieve a higher quality of life. PALS is an evidence-based SM program, evidence based, that surpasses the traditional support group, and is easily adopted by an Amputee Specialty program. PALS SM programs have been shown to reduce depression by 50% over those who attend a regular support group only.[13] PALS programs empower persons with limb loss to learn skills, identify problems early, track their progress so they can participate in their own recovery, and do things to improve their outcomes.

THE PROSTHETIST AND PROSTHETIC INDUSTRY

Each member of the amputee rehabilitation team, if trained well, plays a specific and important role in the care and recovery of the person with limb loss. None is more concrete and pivotal than the prosthetist, but the prosthetist is often the professional outsider on this team of health care providers. Specific efforts must be made to integrate the prosthetist into the team dynamics and maintain this over the course of the life of the amputee.

A first step toward this is for other members of the rehabilitation team gain an understanding of the professional background of prosthetic providers. While the profession lacks national certification standards and significant training and educational variation exists among prosthetists, the industry has been experiencing increased professionalization over the last decade. Today, many prosthetists are trained at a master's level in orthotics and pros- thetics (O&P) and have to complete a clinical internship in orthotics and/or prosthetics and passing a certifying examination. To be eligible to become prosthetist certified, an applicant must provide proper documentation demonstrating graduation from a prosthetist education program accredited by the Commission on Accreditation of Allied Health Education Programs, followed by a prosthetist and/or residency approved by the National Commission on Orthotic and Prosthetic Education. A prosthetist is not necessarily an orthotist or vice versa; each training is specific, with an authoritative examination at the end of a training period. There are 2 certifying bodies in the United States: the American Board for Certification in Orthotics (ABC; www.ABCOP.org) and the Board of Certification/Accreditation, International (BOC; www.BOCUSA.org). Both organizations certify both practitioners and the facilities that provide the services. More than 14,000 O&P practitioners and 7000 facilities are accredited by ABC alone today. Current requirements to receive certification include a degree from an accredited university or college; advanced education at an accredited O&P program; a minimum of 1 year acceptable experience or completion of an accredited residency; and satisfactory completion of written, simulation, and clinical patient management examinations. There are no requirements to be certified in the United States; some individual states require certification and licensure, but many do not. In the health care environment, they go by multiple names: "prosthetists," "orthotists," "CPO" (certified prosthetist orthotist), "providers" (prosthetic/orthotic provider), brace makers, and the condescending "vendors." It is rare that the rest of health care team understands the training, skills, and role of this member of the team, but it is paramount for the success of the person with limb loss that the team develops this understanding and the important professional relationship. As with any member of the health care professional team, a piece of paper, a certificate or license, does not necessarily make a proficient one. The CPO is an artisan, and engineer, a health care provider, and a business professional. As with the rest of the team, they build proficiency with training, education, practice, and oversight. The oversight locally and nationally is marginal; thus, skill levels are variable in the United States. To the person with limb loss and the rest of the team, the gifted CPO is worth his or her weight in gold. A refined socket fit and small adjustments to the prosthetic can mean a huge difference in comfort and tolerance for basic and high-level activity: a skill no other team member brings to the amputee.

FAIR INSURANCE COVERAGE AND NATIONAL ADVOCACY

The Amputee Coalition (www.amputee-coalition.org) is the only national nonprofit advocacy group for persons with limb differences (congenital absence) and limb loss. The Amputee Coalition nationally provides resources and programs to those with limb loss or for those that support them, including health care providers. Their government relations activities include efforts to ensure insurance fairness for lifetime prosthetic coverage. "Parity" is the buzzword meaning "on par with" or "equal to." Legislative parity is the attempt, through either the state or federal legislative process, to seek equalization. In this instance, the legislative parity is specifically health insurance coverage for prosthetics, or prosthetic parity. Prosthetic parity is state or federal legislation requiring insurance companies to pay for prosthetic devices on par with federal programs, payment rules, and regulations. The federal program could be Medicare, Medicaid, or programs such as the federal employee insurance held by Congress and other government employees. These programs provide reimbursement without capitation or exclusions for medically necessary services, such as prosthetic devices.

Not all private insurance policies are created equal. Although many insurances policies do pay for prosthetics without extensive requirements, there is a growing trend across the United States demonstrating that private insurance companies are significantly reducing prosthetic benefits or eliminating prosthetic coverage. The most notable change in prosthetic coverage is the "insurance cap." An insurance cap is a yearly or lifetime benefit maximum. This can be as little as $5000 lifetime coverage, which will not provide the most basic components. These types of caps can be costly and devastating for the new amputee. The cap is a common method used to limit coverage, reducing the company's financial obligation and payout, but still allowing the company to claim to offer the benefit. Yearly caps on prosthetic services range from $500 to $3000, and lifetime restrictions range from $10,000 to 1 prosthetic device during a person's lifetime (from birth to death).

In a recent survey of the 20 major insurance insurers, the number of insurers with financial caps, exclusions, or unusually high deductibles rose 100% during a 6-year period from 2000 to 2006.[48] All 20 insurers surveyed had implemented financial caps to prosthetic coverage. These caps are so important because the cost of 1 lower extremity prosthesis can range in cost from $5000 to $50,000. An upper extremity device or arm can range from $3000 to $30,000. Cost does not define medical appropriateness. An amputee's daily activities, profession, and certain health factors determine the specific materials and technologies used for each custom-manufactured device. Amputation is a catastrophic event with lifelong sequel and needs. Insurance protects against the secondary effects of catastrophic events. That is the expectation on purchasing an insurance policy. It has become increasingly apparent that legislation is necessary to ensure prosthetic coverage and fair payment rules. Through the lobbying efforts of the Amputee Coalition, "arms and legs are not a luxury campaign," federal legislation has been introduced and is working its way through the legislative bodies. In the meantime, they have been successful in 21 states that have passed prosthetic parity legislation over the past 10 years. The legislation is restorative care and would seek to ensure adequate and affordable access to prosthetic devices. The federal legislation would treat external prosthetic devices similar to internal prosthetic devices, like knee and hip replacements, heart stents, and pacemakers, without arbitrary caps and restrictions. The latest insurance battle that seems to be emerging is the new caps on outpatient therapy by CMS that puts the amputee at risk receive appropriate training to meet the potential predicted outcome with the prosthesis.

The Amputee Coalition has been monitoring the implementation of the Affordable Care Act ("Obamacare"), providing comments to the Department of Health and Human Services and to several states regarding the importance of including prosthetic devices in the essential health benefits. Unfortunately, it remains unclear exactly how every benchmark plan will cover prosthetic devices; however, most plans include some level of coverage. They continue to work to communicate the necessity of including prosthetic devices in the essential health benefits under the "Rehabilitative and Habilitative Services and Devices" category. Individuals who pay for insurance through premiums should receive appropriate and medically necessary treatment: their prosthetic arms and legs are not luxury items. Clear messages are voiced that prosthetics provide function, dignity, and self-reliance for those with limb loss.

AMPUTEE MEDICAL HOME

In its landmark 2001 report on Crossing the Quality Chasm, the Institute of Medicine (IOM) named "patient-centered care" as 1 of the 6 fundamental aims of the US health care system.[49] The IOM defines patient-centered care as "Health care that establishes a partnership among practitioners, patients, and their families (when appropriate) to ensure that decisions respect patients' wants, needs, and preferences and that patients have the education and support they need to make decisions and participate in their own care."[50] Interdisciplinary teamwork has shown to improve short-term and long-term outcomes for people with limb loss.[51] With the implementation of the Affordable Care Act, a model of patient-centered and cost-efficient care for specific "groups of patients," known as the medical home, has become a focal point.

The medical home is best described as a model or philosophy of primary care that is patient centered, comprehensive, team based, coordinated, accessible, and focused on quality and safety. It has become a widely accepted model for how primary care should be organized and delivered throughout the health care system, and is a philosophy of health care delivery that encourages providers and care teams to meet

Box 1
Joint principles of the patient-centered medical home

The characteristics of the medical home have been defined within the following 7 principles:

1. Personal physician: Each patient has an ongoing relationship with a personal physician trained to provide first contact, continuous, and comprehensive care.

2. Physician-directed medical practice: The personal physician leads a team of individuals at the practice level who collectively take responsibility for the ongoing care of patients.

3. Whole-person orientation: The personal physician is responsible for providing for all the patient's health care needs or taking responsibility for appropriately arranging care with other qualified professionals. This includes care for all stages of life, acute care, chronic care, preventive services, and end-of-life care.

4. Care is coordinated and/or integrated: Across all elements of the complex health care system (eg, subspecialty care, hospitals, home health agencies, nursing homes) and the patient's community (eg, family, public, and private community-based services). Care is facilitated by registries, information technology, health information exchange, and other means to ensure that patients get the indicated care when and where they need and want it in a culturally and linguistically appropriate manner.

5. Quality and safety are hallmarks of the medical home: Practices advocate for their patients to support the attainment of optimal, patient-centered outcomes that are defined by a care-planning process driven by a compassionate, robust partnership among physicians, patients, and the patient's family.

   • Evidence-based medicine and clinical decision-support tools guide decision making.

   • Physicians in the practice accept accountability for continuous quality improvement through voluntary engagement in performance measurement and improvement.

   • Patients actively participate in decision making, and feedback is sought to ensure patients' expectations are being met.

   • Information technology is used appropriately to support optimal patient care, performance measurement, patient education, and enhanced communication.

   • Practices go through a voluntary recognition process by an appropriate nongovernmental entity to demonstrate that they have the capabilities to provide patient-centered services consistent with the medical home model.

   • Patients and families participate in quality improvement activities at the practice level.

6. Enhanced access to care: Is available through systems such as open scheduling, expanded hours, and new options for communication among patients, their personal physician, and practice staff.

7. Payment: Appropriately recognizes the added value provided to patients who have a patient-centered medical home. The payment structure should be based on the following framework:

   • It should reflect the value of physician and nonphysician staff patient-centered care management work that falls outside of the face-to-face visit.

   • It should pay for services associated with coordination of care both within a given practice and among consultants, ancillary providers, and community resources.

   • It should support adoption and use of health information technology for quality improvement.

   • It should support provision of enhanced communication access, such as secure e-mail and telephone consultation.

   • It should recognize the value of physician work associated with remote monitoring of clinical data using technology.

- It should allow for separate fee-for-service payments for face-to-face visits. (Payments for care management services that fall outside of the face-to-face visit, as described previously, should not result in a reduction in the payments for face-to-face visits.)
- It should recognize case mix differences in the patient population being treated within the practice.
- It should allow physicians to share in savings from reduced hospitalizations associated with physician-guided care management in the office setting.
- It should allow for additional payments for achieving measurable and continuous quality improvements.

Adapted from American Academy of Family Physicians (AAFP), American Academy of Pediatrics (AAP), American College of Physicians (ACP), American Osteopathic Association (AOA). Joint principles of the patient-centered medical home. 2007. Available at: www.acponline.org/pressroom/pcmh.htm.

patients where they are, from the simplest to the most complex conditions. Given the understanding that interdisciplinary team assessment and management should be used in the care of all patients with amputations throughout all phases of care, the medical home is an ideal fit for those with limb loss.

The care of the amputee with special health care needs is the primary focus of the medical home concept. The modern medical home expands on its original foundation, becoming a home base for any amputee's medical and nonmedical care. Ideally, the person should be transferred to a specialty program devoted exclusively to the care of amputees as soon as possible after amputation. Receiving inpatient rehabilitation immediately after acute care improves survival rates, reduces subsequent amputations, and correlates with greater acquisition of prosthetic devices and greater medical stability than for patients who are sent home or to a skilled nursing facility.[52] This becomes the entry into the amputee medical home, where the person receives concerted care coordination and navigation by an accountable team available for all lifetime needs. Above all, the medical home is not a final destination, instead it is a model for achieving amputee care excellence so that care is received in the right place, at the right time, and in the manner that best suits an amputee's needs. Today's medical home is a cultivated partnership among the patient, family/supports, and primary provider in cooperation with specialists, prosthetists, therapists, case managers, social workers, and support from the community. The patient/family is the focal point of this model, and the medical home is built around this center. Family members of amputees play a critical role in the entire treatment process, including the establishment of short-term and long-term goals. We learned from our military limb loss experts that education and training for family caregivers is an integral part of the care of the combat amputee.[53] Basic guidelines stress that care under the medical home model must be accessible, person centered, continuous, comprehensive, coordinated, compassionate, and culturally effective. The amputee home model should reflect the Joint Principles of the Patient-Centered Medical Home as developed collaboratively in 2007 by the AAP joined with the American Academy of Family Physicians, the American College of Physicians, and the American Osteopathic Association (**Box 1**).

ACKNOWLEDGMENTS

With appreciation to Marya Sabalbaro, BS, for her tireless organizational and administrative support.

REFERENCES

1. Zeigler-Graham K, MacKenzie E, Ephraim P, et al. Estimating the prevalence of limb loss in the United States 2005 to 2050. Arch Phys Med Rehabil 2008;89(3): 422–9.
2. HCUPnet. Healthcare Cost and Utilization Project. Nationwide Inpatient Sample (NIS). Rockville (MD): Agency for Healthcare Research and Quality. Accessed May 28, 2013.
3. Mackenzie E, Jones A, Bosse M, et al. Health-care costs associated with amputation or reconstruction of a limb threatening injury. J Bone Joint Surg Am 2007; 89(8):1685–92.
4. Alemayehu B, Warner K. The lifetime distribution of healthcare costs. Health Services Research 2004;39(3):627–42.
5. Blough D, Hubbard S, McFarland L, et al. Prosthetic costs projections for service members with major limb loss from Vietnam and OIF/OEF. J Rehabil Res Dev 2010;47(4):387–402.
6. Naschitz J, Lenger R. Why traumatic leg amputees are at increased risk for cardiovascular disease. QJM 2008;101(4):251–9.
7. Kurdibylo E. Obesity and metabolic orders in adults with lower limb amputation. J Rehabil Res Dev 1996;33(4):387–94.
8. Gailey R, Allen K, Castles J, et al. Review of secondary physical conditions associated with lower-limb amputation and long term prosthetic use. J Rehabil Res Dev 2008;45(1):15–30.
9. Coffey L, Gallagher P, Horogan O, et al. Psychosocial adjustment to diabetes related lower limb amputation. Diabet Med 2009;26(10):1063–7.
10. Veterans Health Administration. Preservation—amputation care and treatment (PACT) program. Washington, DC: Department of Veterans Affairs; 2006.
11. Schoefield C, Libby G, Brennan G, et al. Mortality and hospitalization in patients after amputation. Diabetes Care 2006;29(10):2252–6.
12. Barmparas G, Inaba K, Teixeria P, et al. Epidemiology of post-traumatic limb amputation: a national trauma databank analysis. Am Surg 2010;76(11):1214–22.
13. Wegener S, Mackenzie EJ, Ephraim P, et al. Self management improves outcomes in persons with limb loss. Arch Phys Med Rehabil 2009;90(3):373–80.
14. Selvin E, Erlinger T. Prevalence of and risk factors for peripheral arterial disease in the United States: results from the National Health and Nutrition Examination Survey. Circulation 2004;110(6):738–43.
15. Melton PA. Peripheral vascular disease and diabetes. Diabetes in America (2), 12. 2002.
16. Dillingham TR, Pezzin LE, MacKenzie EJ. Limb amputation and limb deficiency: epidemiology and recent trends in the United States. South Med J 2002;95(8): 875–83.
17. Gloviczki P. Revascularization decreases amputation by 40% in patients with PAD. Society of Vascular Surgery Annual meeting. San Francisco (CA), May 30–June 1, 2013.
18. Canavan R, Unwin N, Kelly W, et al. Diabetes and non diabetes related lower extremity amputation incidence before and after the introduction of better organized diabetes foot care: continuous longitudinal monitoring using a standard method. Diabetes Care 2008;31:459–63.
19. Li Y, Burrow N, Gregg E, et al. Declining rates of hospitalization for nontraumatic lower extremity amputation in the diabetic population aged 40 years or older: US 1988-2008. Diabetes Care 2012;35:273–7.

20. Margolis DJ, Hoffstad O, Nafash J, et al. Location, location, location: geographic clustering of lower-extremity amputation among Medicare beneficiaries with diabetes. Diabetes Care 2011;34:2363–7.
21. Flegal KM, Carroll MD, Kit BK, et al. Prevalence of obesity and trends in the distribution of body mass index among US adults, 1999-2010. JAMA 2012;307(5): 491–7.
22. Levi J, Segal L, et al. F as in fat: how obesity threatens America's future. Washington DC: Trust for America's Health (TFAH); 2012.
23. Sohn M, Budiman-Mak E, Lee T, et al. Significant J-shaped association between body mass index (BMI) and diabetic foot ulcers. Diabetes Metab Res Rev 2011; 27(4):402–9.
24. Resnick H, Carter E, Sosenko J, et al. Incidence of lower-extremity amputation in American Indians: the Strong Heart Study. Diabetes Care 2004; 27(8):1885–91.
25. Kalbaugh C, Taylor S, Kalbaugh B, et al. Does obesity predict functional outcome in dysvascular amputees? Am Surg 2006;72(8):707–13.
26. Richardson L, Irvin C, Tamayo-Sarver J, et al. Racial and ethnic disparities in the clinical practice of emergency medicine. Acad Emerg Med 2003;10:1184–8.
27. Lantz P, Lynch J, House J, et al. Socioeconomic disparities in health change in a longitudinal study of US adults: the role of health-risk behaviors. Soc Sci Med 2006;53(1):167–75.
28. Oster N, Welch V, Schild L, et al. Differences in self management behaviors and use of preventative services among diabetes management enrollees by race and ethnicity. Dis Manag 2006;9(3):167–75.
29. Holman K, Henke P, Dimick J, et al. Racial disparities in the use of revascularization before leg amputation in Medicare patients. J Vasc Surg 2011;52(2):420–6.
30. Lefebre K, Lavery L. Disparities in amputations in minorities. Clin Orthop Relat Res 2011;469(7):1941–50.
31. Dillingham T, Pezzin L, MacKenzie E, et al. Racial differences in the incidence of limb loss secondary to peripheral vascular disease; a population based study. Arch Phys Med Rehabil 2002;83:1252–7.
32. Eslami M, Zayaruzny M, Fitzgerald G, et al. The adverse effects of race, insurance status, and low income on the rate of amputation in patients presenting with lower extremity ischemia. J Vasc Surg 2007;45(1):55.
33. Regenbogen S, Gawande A, Lipsitz SR, et al. Do differences in hospital and surgeon quality explain racial disparities in lower-extremity vascular amputation? Am Surg 2009;250(3):424–31.
34. Indian Health Service. Trends in Indian Health. Bethesda (MD): US Department of Health and Human Services; 2004.
35. O'Connell J, Yi R, Wilson C, et al. Racial disparities in health status: a comparison of the morbidity among American Indian and US adults with diabetes. Diabetes Care 2010;33(7):1463–70.
36. National Center for Health Statistics. Number in thousands of hospital discharges for non-traumatic lower extremity amputation with diabetes as a listed diagnosis. CDC; 2012. Available at: www.cdc.gov/diabetis/statistics/lea/fig1.html. Accessed July 2013.
37. Murphy S, Xu J, Kochanek K. Deaths: preliminary data for 2100. Washington, DC: CDC; 2002.
38. Haas LB, Ahroni JH. Lower limb self management education. In: Bowker JH, Pfeifer MA, editors. The Diabetic Foot. Philadelphia: Mosby-Elsevier; 2001. p. 665–75.

39. Pecaro R, Reiber G, Burges E. Pathway to diabetic limb amputation: basis for prevention. Diabetes Care 1990;13(5):513–21.
40. Ortegon M, Redekop W, Niessen L. Cost effectiveness of prevention and treatment of the diabetic foot. Diabetes Care 2010;27(4):901–7.
41. Roberts TL, Pasquina PF, Nelson VS. Limb deficiencies and prosthetic management. 4. Comorbidities associated with limb loss. Arch Phys Med Rehabil 2006; 87(3 Suppl 1):S21–7.
42. McCollum P, Raza Z. Vascular disease: limb salvage versus amputation. In: Atlas of Amputations and LImb Deficiencies. Rosemont, IL: American Academy of Orthopaedic Surgeons; 2004. 31.
43. Archdeacon MT, Sanders R. Trauma: limb salvage versus amputation. In: Atlas of Amputations and LImb Deficiencies. Rosemont, IL: American Academy of Orthopaedic Surgeons; 2004. p. 69–74.
44. Nelson VS, Flood KM, Bryant PR, et al. Limb Deficiency and prosthetic management; 1: decision making in prosthetic prescription and management. Arch Phys Med Rehabil 2006;87(3 Suppl 1):S3–9.
45. Darnal B, Ephraim PW, Dillingham T, et al. Depressive symptoms and mental health services utilization among persons with limb loss: results of a national survey. Arch Phys Med Rehabil 2005;86(4):650–8.
46. Ephraim P, Wegener S, MacKenzie E, et al. Phantom pain, residual limb pain, and back pain in amputees. Arch Phys Med Rehabil 2005;86(10):1910–9.
47. Marincek B. Return to work after lower limb amputation. Disabil Rehabil 2007; 29(17):1323–9.
48. Turner R. Article source: prosthetic parity—what is it? 2007. Available at: http://EzineArticles.com/645273.
49. Institute of Medicine. Crossing the quality chasm: a new health system for 21st century. Washington, DC: National Academy Press; 2001.
50. Institute of Medicine. Envisioning the national health care quality report. Washington DC: National Academy Press; 2001.
51. Pasquina P. Advances in amputee care. Arch Phys Med Rehabil 2006; 87(3 Suppl 1):534–43.
52. Dillingham TR, Pezzin LE. Rehabilitation setting and associated mortality and medical stability among persons with amputation.
53. Pasquina P, Cooper R. Care of the combat amputee. Falls Church, VA: Office of the Surgeon General; 2010.

Principles of Contemporary Amputation Rehabilitation in the United States, 2013

Robert H. Meier III, MD[a],*, Jeffrey T. Heckman, DO[b]

KEYWORDS

- Amputation • Rehabilitation • Veterans Health Administration • Follow-up care

KEY POINTS

- Providing rehabilitation services for the person with an amputation has become more difficult in today's health care environment.
- Amputation rehabilitation calls for specialized, multidisciplinary rehabilitation training.
- In examining the principles of amputation rehabilitation, one must understand the lessons learned from the Veterans Affairs Amputation System of Care and return to the founding principles of rehabilitation medicine.
- Persons with amputations must be reevaluated in a tight program of follow-up care.

Physiatric management for persons with limb loss remains a nascent subspecialty in physical medicine and rehabilitation, with only 2 fellowship opportunities in the country.[1–5] The cause of limb loss and diversity of patient population make this a challenging area to gain expertise during brief periods of training during a physiatrist's residency education. In addition, services available to civilians with limb loss in the private world vary greatly from those for veterans or active service members with limb loss in the United States. Therefore, as physiatrists caring for persons with limb loss in both the civilian sector and the Veterans Health Administration (VHA), the authors review current principles of amputation rehabilitation medicine within these health care systems.

PRINCIPLES OF AMPUTATION REHABILITATION FOR THE CIVILIAN WITH LIMB LOSS

Providing rehabilitation services for the person with an amputation has become more difficult in today's health care environment. This increased difficulty has occurred

[a] Amputee Services of America, Denver, CO, USA; [b] Department of Rehabilitation Medicine, Regional Amputation Center (RAC), VA Puget Sound Health Care System, Seattle Division, University of Washington, 1660 South Columbian Way, Seattle, WA 98108, USA
* Corresponding author.
E-mail address: skipdoc3@gmail.com

Phys Med Rehabil Clin N Am 25 (2014) 29–33
http://dx.doi.org/10.1016/j.pmr.2013.09.004
1047-9651/14/$ – see front matter © 2014 Elsevier Inc. All rights reserved.

because of a confluence of factors that are involved in an amputation, the person undergoing an amputation, health care reimbursement, changes in methods of providing rehabilitation services, the availability of new technology, and changes in professional discipline attitudes toward rehabilitation. In fact, the actual definition of rehabilitation should be challenged in today's environment.

Previously, rehabilitation was neatly defined as a team effort to restore meaningful function. Currently, amputee rehabilitation is often defined as placing a prosthesis on the amputee, without particular measurement of the outcome achieved by providing the prosthesis. In addition, the prosthesis is often provided by a physician signing a prescription that has been developed by a prosthetist. Thus, in some settings, amputation rehabilitation has been reduced to involving only the patient, the surgeon, and the prosthetist. This trio may not end up with a satisfactory functional result, and really ignores the emotional adaptation to the loss of a limb and its psychosocial consequences. This trio may also not embody the experience or knowledge to address the complex issues of pain, whether acute or chronic.

The period of inpatient rehabilitation has almost disappeared in many locations in the United States. If it is provided, it is focused on mobility function before the fitting of the prosthesis. A period of inpatient or outpatient rehabilitation once the prosthesis is obtained often does not occur in a team setting. Many amputees are trained in the home setting by home-based therapists who may not have much experience with training the amputee in the technology used in the prosthesis. In addition, this method of prosthetic training does not avail itself of the traditional rehabilitation treatment team (ie, amputee, rehabilitation physician, physical therapist, occupational therapist, and psychosocial counselor, at a minimum) to provide comprehensive rehabilitation services. In addition, many inpatient rehabilitation settings are not set up to provide comprehensive rehabilitation services that include the health professionals traditionally included in the rehabilitation treatment team.

Furthermore, therapy services are now rationed for patients sponsored by Medicare and some private health insurance providers. The number of outpatient therapy visits may be limited. In some cases, the therapy visits have been incorporated into the pre-prosthetic phase, and the number of visits available is insufficient for proper prosthetic training. It has become incumbent on the rehabilitation team to determine how best to use the limited number of therapy visits for the most optimal functional outcome. This management requires careful forethought and planning by the rehabilitation team before therapeutic services are instituted.

Another issue seen in today's mish mash of what is called rehabilitation is that team members may not understand what the desirable outcome should be. This uncertainty may result from a lack of training, experience, knowledge, or team coordination. Often, the amputee is not told early in the rehabilitation experience what the objectively measureable goals should be and how much time it will take to achieve these goals. Thus, some amputees are not guided to the point of excellent prosthetic function because the therapist, prosthetist, and perhaps even treating physician do not know what the end goal could and should be.

Amputation rehabilitation really calls for specialized, multidisciplinary rehabilitation training. So many new prosthetic designs and technologically advanced, expensive prosthetic components are now available, and therapists, physicians, and prosthetists with experience in training the amputee should be involved in this process. Some prosthetic component manufacturers tout new components as having the supposed advantage that the amputee will need less therapy to learn to use the device. What often happens is that these technologic advances require the same amount or more therapy to get the best result from these newer and more expensive components.

Although keeping up with the many prosthetic advances and changes is difficult, it is important for physiatrists to keep abreast of the latest developments if they are going to sign prescriptions for these devices. The claims for improved function from some of the new technology have not been objectively studied, and often no data are available to suggest that the added expense is warranted. Furthermore, often the hidden motive is that the prosthetist, physician, or therapist wishes to try the newest components at someone else's expense. With all of this new technology, it is important for the rehabilitation physician to read prosthetic journals and attend the professional shows for the orthotists and prosthetists.

In addition, physicians who sign the prescriptions must know what they are prescribing, just as they would with a medication. Knowing what the prosthetic prescription will cost in usual and customary dollars is also important. A more even-handed way to keep track of prosthetic costs is to know what the Medicare allowable amount will be for a particular set of "L" codes.

PRINCIPLES OF AMPUTATION REHABILITATION FOR THE VETERAN WITH LIMB LOSS

The VHA has developed the model for an integrated system in which Veterans Affairs (VA) physicians, therapists, and prosthetists work together to provide specialized expertise in amputation care incorporating the latest practices in medical rehabilitation, therapy services, and prosthetic technology. Developed in the early part of the 21st century, the system was implemented in 2008 to enhance the environment of care and ensure consistency in the delivery of rehabilitation services for veterans with limb loss. The VA Amputation System of Care (ASoC) provides support for salary, training, education, travel, and equipment to allow VA professionals the ability to provide veterans with the most advanced technology and state-of-the-art care. This system provides care through more than 375,000 clinical visits to more than 30,000 veterans with limb loss, including more than 1300 veterans from Operations Enduring Freedom, Iraqi Freedom, and New Dawn.

The ASoC consists of 4 levels of care. Seven Regional Amputation Centers provide comprehensive rehabilitation care through an interdisciplinary team and serve as resources across the system through the use of telerehabilitation technologies. These centers provide the highest level of specialized expertise in clinical care and technology, and provide rehabilitation and consultation to patients with the most complex conditions. The 7 locations are Bronx, NY; Denver, CO; Minneapolis, MN; Palo Alto, CA; Richmond, VA; Seattle, WA; and Tampa, FL. Eighteen Polytrauma/Amputation Network Sites provide a full range of clinical and ancillary services to veterans closer to home. A total of 108 Amputation Clinic Teams provide specialized outpatient amputation care, and 22 Amputation Points of Contact facilitate referrals and access to services.

The organizational structure of the ASoC strives to provide ease of access to high-quality care for veterans with limb loss. A focus on virtual care using telemedicine equipment allows Regional Amputation Centers to connect with veterans with limb loss in rural areas to provide specialized clinical decision making and prosthesis prescription writing. With a detailed prosthesis prescription, all enrolled veterans may receive any prosthetic item prescribed by a VA clinician, without regard to service connection, when it is determined to promote, preserve, or restore the health of the individual and is in accord with generally accepted standards of medical practice.

A dedication and commitment to education and advancing research is apparent within the ASoC working collaboratively with the VA Research and Development Centers of Excellence in Limb Loss Prevention and Prosthetic Engineering and joint VA/Department of Defense programs (ie, Extremity Trauma and Amputation Center of Excellence). To date, the ASoC has published the "Clinical Practice Guidelines for Rehabilitation of Lower Limb Amputation: a Clinician Toolkit," focusing on pain management, management of the residual limb, and analysis and treatment of abnormal gait, and a patient-focused publication titled *The Next Step: The Rehabilitation Journey After Lower Limb Amputation*.[6,7] In addition, the "Clinical Practice Guideline Following Upper Limb Amputation" is expected to publish in 2014.[8]

MULTIDISCIPLINARY APPROACH

The patient population evaluated by the ASoC has similar causes of amputation as the general population, with the most likely cause for amputation surgery being vascular disease related to diabetes mellitus type 2. These patients require an interdisciplinary approach, including vascular surgery, orthopedic surgery, wound care, nursing, primary care, podiatry, endocrinology, infectious disease, rehabilitation medicine, physical and occupational therapy, psychology, social work, and prosthetics services. The VA has developed a collaborative program integrating these various disciplines, called Prevention of Amputation for Veterans Everywhere (PAVE), which is coordinated locally at each facility. The PAVE program and the ASoC are closely linked and coordinate efforts to address the prevention of primary and secondary amputation. Each member of the multidisciplinary team caring for veterans at risk for amputation has a specific role along the continuum of care.

In examining the principles of amputation rehabilitation, one must understand the lessons learned from the ASoC and return to the founding principles of rehabilitation medicine. Following are several of the foundation principles for this disability, some of which of course overlap with other areas of disability:

1. The amputee is the most important member of the team.
2. Amputation rehabilitation requires a multidisciplinary team, which often includes the patient, a surgeon, a rehabilitation physician, a physical therapist, an occupational therapist, a psychosocial counselor, and a prosthetist, at a minimum. Other health professionals and specialists may also have important roles in this integrated team. Often, a case manager from the hospital and/or the third-party payer should be an integral team member.
3. The rehabilitation process should be predominantly one of education. Through education, amputees become empowered to take control of their future lives and make decisions based on complete information.
4. Amputees can be further empowered if they are educated about what the expectations of function and emotional well-being are likely to be once the early program of rehabilitation is completed. It is crucial that amputees know what can be accomplished under the best of circumstances, both with and without use of a prosthesis.
5. Amputation rehabilitation is a process, and must unfold with careful guidance from experienced rehabilitation professionals.
6. Based on the functional goals of the amputee, the rehabilitation team should consider how the amputee will ideally be functioning at 1 year, 5 years, 10 years, and later throughout life. The amputation is a permanent disability and should be considered through the decades of life, not just in the initial phases of rehabilitation.
7. After amputation, the motivation to wear a prosthesis varies based on many factors. Therefore, the rehabilitation approach must focus on function as the prevailing mission based on the patient's goals, and should not be limited to the use of a prosthesis.

8. An important aspect of rehabilitation for the person with an amputation is their psychosocial adaptation to the amputation and the changes that accompany the loss of a body part.
9. Fabrication and application of a prosthesis for an amputee is universal. The goal of amputation rehabilitation is to help the amputee move forward in life and regain good quality of life, with or without a prosthesis.
10. Amputation rehabilitation is a lifelong process requiring continuity of care for rehabilitation services and prosthesis management. This long-term approach permits measurement of physical and emotional outcomes reflecting the value of the acute rehabilitation process.

There is no one right or wrong way to deliver comprehensive rehabilitation services. Each setting must define what amputation rehabilitation means and establish a system that fulfills that definition. Little question exists that a complete rehabilitation program will require both inpatient and outpatient phases. Discussion with the referring surgeons about the rehabilitation program that is envisioned will assist them in becoming integrated members of the whole rehabilitation treatment team. The rehabilitation doctor must understand when the surgeon is willing to have the rehabilitation doctor assume most of the health care decisions for the amputee.

Persons with an amputation must be reevaluated in a tight program of follow-up care, which means that they should have regular and periodic follow-up appointments, and understand why these appointments are important for their continuing care. Follow-up care permits the team to assess the fit of the prosthesis, the function achieved, ability to return to work, mechanical problems with the prosthesis, pain issues, and the patient's emotional well-being, overall health, and perceived quality of life. This follow-up should be a regular and lifelong process. This plan of care does not make the amputee dependent on the health care system, but serves more as a preventive strategy to address the particular needs of persons with an amputation.

REFERENCES

1. Meier RH, Esquenazi A. Rehabilitation planning for the upper extremity amputee. In: Meier RH, Atkins DJ, editors. Functional restoration of adults and children with upper extremity amputation. New York: Demos Medical; 2004.
2. Meier RH. Amputations and prosthetic fitting. In: Fisher SV, Helm PA, editors. Comprehensive rehabilitation of burns. Baltimore (MD): Williams & Wilkins; 1984.
3. Leonard JA, Meier RH. Upper and lower extremity prosthetics. In: DeLisa JA, Gans BM, editors. Rehabilitation medicine principles and practice. 3rd edition. Lippincott Raven; 1998.
4. Meier RH. Rehabilitation of the person with an amputation. In: Rutherford RB, editor. Vascular surgery. 4th edition. Philadelphia: WB Saunders Company; 1995.
5. Available at: http://www.aapmr.org/career/fellowshipdb. Accessed October 22, 2013.
6. ASoC. VA/DoD Clinical Practice Guidelines for Rehabilitation of Lower Limb Amputation: Clinician Tool Kit. Available at: http://www.healthquality.va.gov/Lower_Limb_Amputation.asp. 2008. Accessed October 23, 2013.
7. ASoC. The Next Step: The Rehabilitation Journey After Lower Limb Amputation. Available at: https://www.qmo.amedd.army.mil/amp/Handbook.pdf. 2008. Accessed October 23, 2013.
8. ASoC. VA/DoD Clinical Practice Guidelines for Rehabilitation of Lower Limb Amputation. Available at: http://www.healthquality.va.gov/Lower_Limb_Amputation.asp. Accessed October 23, 2013.

Amputation Surgery

David Schnur, MD[a], Robert H. Meier III, MD[b],*

KEYWORDS

- Amputation • Osseointegrated implant • Targeted muscle reinnervation • Allograft

KEY POINTS

- There are instances when stump revision should be considered to provide a better prosthetic fitting and function.
- The best level of amputation must take into consideration the newest socket designs, methods of prosthetic suspension, and technologically advanced components.
- Targeted reinnervation is a new neural-machine interface that has been developed to help improve the function of electrically powered upper prosthetic limbs.
- Osseointegrated implants for prosthetic suspension offer amputees an alternative to the traditional socket suspension, and are especially useful for transfemoral and transhumeral levels of amputation.
- Cadaver bone can be used to lengthen an extremely short residual bony lever arm.

INTRODUCTION AND PHILOSOPHY OF AMPUTATION SURGERY

Amputation surgery should always be viewed as reconstructive surgery, with the thought that the amputated extremity will provide less pain and better function than the limb would have if it had not been amputated.

Included in the goals of amputation surgery should be:

1. Remove nonviable, diseased, or infected tissues
2. Provide a residual limb that will be useful for prosthetic function
3. Cover the residual limb with full-thickness soft tissue including muscle and fascia covering the bone
4. Taper the ends of the bone without sharp or rough edges
5. Provide a cylindrically shaped residual limb that provides a better prosthetic fit than a conically shaped limb
6. Primary wound healing within 3 to 5 weeks
7. Control of postsurgical edema
8. No hematoma formation

[a] Plastic Surgery Clinic of Denver, Humboldt Street, Denver, CO 80218, USA; [b] Amputee Services of America, East 19th Avenue, Denver, CO 80218, USA
* Corresponding author.
E-mail address: skipdoc3@gmail.com

Phys Med Rehabil Clin N Am 25 (2014) 35–43
http://dx.doi.org/10.1016/j.pmr.2013.09.013
1047-9651/14/$ – see front matter © 2014 Elsevier Inc. All rights reserved.

9. Gentle handling and retraction of the nerves up into the stump
10. Preservation of length that will accommodate contemporary prosthetic components
11. Excellent postoperative pain control

Surgical techniques to achieve these goals are covered in other surgical texts noted in the Selected Readings at the conclusion of this article. However, a few of the newer surgical options are mentioned here. Increasing in popularity for the below-knee amputee is the Ertl procedure, which is categorized as an osteoplasty. For the below-knee amputee, a piece of autologous bone is placed between the ends of the tibia and fibula, secured in place and permitted to solidly fuse in place. This procedure usually results in a more cylindrically shaped residual leg that is considered to permit better fitting of the prosthetic socket, and often can take direct end pressure on the stump.

Another newer technique now available to salvage a limb or to provide longer length is the use of allograft (cadaver) bone. If there is inadequate tissue to cover the increased bone length, full-thickness flap surgery can be used to cover the new bone length. Often this can add an additional 3 to 4 inches (7.5–10 cm) of bone length that can make a significant difference in the lever arm available to move the prosthesis, especially if the starting residual limb is very short.

A surgery used in Sweden and being investigated in the United States is called osseous integration, or direct skeletal attachment. A female coupling device is inserted into the residual bone and held in place with cement. The exoskeletal prosthesis is then attached using a male coupler that is the proximal end of the prosthesis. With this secure coupling, no socket is needed for the residual limb. With this design, all movement of the bones of the residual limb is directly transferred to motoring the prosthetic components. One disadvantage of this process is that as yet, no material has been found into which the skin will heal and provide a bacterial barrier. In some cases, infection has become a chronic problem and the long-term use of antibiotics has been necessary. In a few cases, the residual limb has fractured above the inserted female component, which then needs to be removed.

Free bone grafts have become useful in preserving all available length of the residual limb. These grafts are autografts, and can be taken from a fibula or a scapular margin.

Targeted muscle reinnervation (TMR) is being used in a few centers to create new muscle signals for myoelectric control. This procedure is often used in proximal levels of arm amputation where few muscles remain from which to obtain muscle signal sites.

Postoperative techniques to protect the residual limb incision include a variety of methods:

1. Rigid postoperative casting
2. Rigid removable cast
3. Immediate-fit prosthesis
4. Soft, bulky dressing

Each of these techniques has its advantages and disadvantages. The best technique is probably the one agreed upon by the amputation team, the pros and cons of which are understood by the team. No one technique has been shown to improve the eventual outcome of wound healing or prosthetic use, or to lessen the costs of health care.

Covering the residual bones with muscle, fascia, and full-thickness skin provides the most durable covering for the constant pounding of the residual limb from prosthetic function. In addition, a scar that is mobile over the bones of the residual limb decreases shearing forces on the skin when the prosthesis is worn and used functionally.

STUMP REVISION

There are instances whereby stump revision should be considered to provide a better prosthetic fitting and function. The following is a list of circumstances whereby revision should be considered and discussed with the rehabilitation team, as different team members may observe different issues regarding the residual limb and prosthetic fitting.

1. Sharp bony edges that are painful inside the prosthetic socket
2. A palpable neuroma that is symptomatic, or a neuroma, seen on magnetic resonance imaging, that is painful
3. Inadequate soft-tissue coverage to permit excellent prosthetic wearing over several years remaining in life
4. Need for additional residual limb length
5. Floppy long bone in the residual limb soft tissue so that the transmission of forces to the prosthetic socket are decreased. This feature may be secondary to the lack of a myoplastic or myodesis closure or, in addition, the myoplasty or myodesis may have come apart so that the residual long bone is not anchored in the surrounding soft tissues
6. The presence of heterotopic bone formation that interferes with comfortable socket wearing, or important joint motion that produces essential prosthetic function
7. Inadequate soft-tissue coverage or poor residual limb contouring
8. Scar that is adherent to the underlying tissues
9. Symptomatic neuroma formation

CONTROVERSIAL LEVELS OF AMPUTATION

It is possible that some surgeons will disagree on everything that is stated here. However, the best level of amputation must take into consideration the newest socket designs, methods of prosthetic suspension, and technologically advanced components. Often, the crucial factor in this area of debate is the length of the residual limb. When one considers the length of the residual limb, it must include not just the bony length but the length to the end of the soft tissues covering the bone.

Some levels that commonly create limitations in prosthetic fitting and use of components are:

1. Any very short level of amputation; this makes leverage of the prosthesis difficult and provides a smaller surface area over which to distribute the forces require for efficient prosthetic function
2. Disarticulations of the elbow, wrist, knee, and ankle
3. Very long levels of the residual humerus, radius, and ulna
4. Very long levels of the femur, tibia, and fibula

A disarticulation level of amputation results in bony prominences at the end of the residual limb that require a distal prosthetic socket larger than would be necessary if a shorter amputation had been performed, whereby the bony prominences had been removed. The distal dimensions of the disarticulation socket can be cosmetically unsatisfactory and quite bulky. Moreover, there may only be full-thickness skin covering these bony prominences, making prosthetic wearing less comfortable than if the prominence were removed and the stump covered with a myoplasty.

Most disarticulation levels also limit the prosthetic components that can be used, and some of the newest prosthetic technology cannot be used in a disarticulation level of prosthesis.

On average, to use contemporary prosthetic components for a transhumeral prosthesis, 7.6 cm of space above the elbow center is required so that the prosthetic elbow center is at the level of the intact elbow. In the transfemoral amputee, 10.2 cm are necessary above the knee axis to use today's microprocessor knees and keep the knee axis at an equal level to the intact leg (**Figs. 1** and **2**).

For the below-knee amputee, 17.7 cm are required from the floor to the ends of the amputated limb soft tissues to enable use of the newer microprocessor foot/ankle complexes.

However, some of the disarticulation levels have distinct advantages. At the above-elbow level, rotational control of the prosthesis is improved relative to a standard level of above-elbow amputation. Another advantage is the ability to keep the proximal trim lines of the socket lower on the proximal humerus. In addition, the residual internal and external rotation of the humerus can be transmitted to the socket, improving placement of the terminal device.

For the wrist disarticulation level, again the proximal prosthetic socket trim lines can be kept lower on the residual forearm. Moreover, the prominences of the radius and ulna can permit a socket design that is self-suspending.

At the knee disarticulation level, the above-knee socket is less likely to rotate on the residual leg, suspension is easier in the prosthetic socket, and there can often be direct end bearing inside the socket.

An ankle disarticulation is a Syme level of leg amputation and with a stable and full-thickness heel pad can permit end bearing for the person to walk without needing to don a prosthetic leg. Moreover, the proximal trim lines can be kept lower on the socket, and socket suspension is easier than with a traditional-length below-knee amputation.

Skillful revision of an amputation stump is an important aspect of the amputation surgeon's expertise. Many times, amputations are performed in less than ideal conditions. Trauma or marginal vascularity can compromise tissues and negatively affect results of an amputation. Other times, amputations are performed by surgeons who are not as skilled in the nuances of amputation surgery, which may lead to a

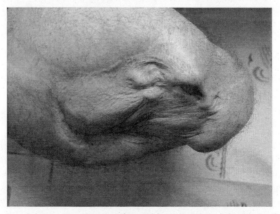

Fig. 1. A young man with traumatic transfemoral amputation developed heterotopic bone that prevents wearing a prosthesis because of pain in the socket.

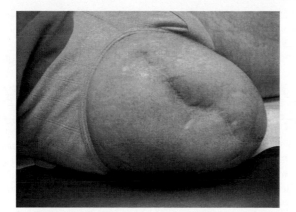

Fig. 2. Transfemoral residual leg of the patient in **Fig. 1** following revision surgery. Following revision surgery, heterotopic bone removal permits comfortable wearing.

suboptimal stump. Occasionally, amputations are done well by skilled surgeons but complications such as infection, hematoma, or dehiscence leave a stump that can be problematic. Often the suboptimal stump can be transformed into a very functional stump with a properly planned and executed revisional procedure. At their institution the authors take a multidisciplinary approach to these challenges with physical medicine specialists, orthopedic surgeons, plastic surgeons, and prosthetists all working together to maximize the benefits of these procedures.

Indications for amputation revision generally fall into 2 main categories, the first of which is improvement of the physical attributes of the stump to make the patient a better prosthetic wearer. The second category is treatment of the painful stump, a more difficult endeavor that must have clear indications and goals to be successful.

Regarding the physical attributes of the stump, improving the soft-tissue envelope of the stump is the most common indication for revision surgery, which is especially true for the below-knee amputation. For the most part this description focuses on the transtibial stump as it pertains to revision surgery. Often patients will present with a stump that has excess soft tissue. During primary amputations, surgeons are careful to leave adequate soft tissue for the stump, but occasionally overestimate the amount of soft tissue that is necessary. In addition, an amputation may be performed on a swollen extremity, and once the swelling subsides the stump is left with an abundant soft-tissue envelope. These revisional procedures are probably the simplest. In these cases, the old scar is typically excised and the incision can be extended to facilitate skin removal. Dissection is carried down to the fascia with Bovie cautery under tourniquet control if possible. Skin and fat flaps are elevated both anteriorly and posteriorly, with more limited dissection on the anterior surface. If muscle is to be debulked then the fascia is divided toward the anterior aspect of the tibia. Dissection is carried out down to the tibia, and muscle can be elevated off of the bone. At this point, the muscle can be debulked and, if necessary, can be debulked in the coronal plane. If both the soleus and the gracilis muscle have been rotated, the soleus can be excised proximal to the bone and the gracilis can be rerotated over the tibia. If there is excess bulk with a single muscle belly, one should not hesitate to divide this in the coronal plane and rerotate the muscle. If some bony revision is necessary, such as excising an exostosis, it can be done at this point. Also, the surgeon should ensure that the tibia has been adequately beveled anteriorly and, if not the case, this can be done at this time. The muscle is then secured over the tibia with either a myodesis or myoplasty. The most common practice, especially when the muscle has slid off of the tibia, is to secure it to the bone with drill holes through the anterior cortex, typically done with an 0 PDS suture. A second layer of running 2-0 Vicryl is then used to secure the posterior muscle to the anterior muscle bellies and fascia.

At this point, the tourniquet is deflated and careful hemostasis is obtained with the Bovie cautery. A 10-mm flat Jackson-Pratt drain is then placed to ensure that fluid does not collect under the skin flap. This step is an important one, and should not be skipped. Next, the skin is trimmed to ensure a snug but not overly tight closure; the skin excision should be designed to enhance the shape of the stump, giving it a conical shape. Dermal sutures are place with 3-0 Monocryl and the skin is closed with 3-0 nylon in interrupted vertical mattress fashion. The authors then place a dressing with antibiotic ointment, Xeroform, and gauze, with a Kerlix wrap and ace wraps in figure-of-8 fashion.

Postoperatively, the drain is removed when the output is less than 30 mL of fluid per 24-hour period. The sutures are left in for 2 weeks, at which point a formal stump shrinker is applied. The stump is then non–weight bearing for a full 6 weeks. At this point, the prosthetist must carefully evaluate the new stump to assess if a new socket is warranted. In most circumstances this is true, so the stump can be cast at 5 to 6 weeks for the new socket.

The more difficult revision is the scenario of soft-tissue paucity on the stump, which can lead to pain, soft-tissue breakdown, or both. In this situation it is important to assess the bony length of the stump and to determine whether shortening bone length to gain a relative soft-tissue increase is possible. At the below-knee amputation level, stumps with as little as 5 cm of tibia can be fitted by the adroit prosthetist. The authors have seen patients fitted with shorter stumps; however, this becomes very difficult for even the most skilled prosthetist.

If shortening is an option, many of the same surgical steps for the revision surgery are similar. The posterior muscle may need to be released more in this case and then rotated over the shortened tibia and fibula. Fixation of the muscle and closure proceed in a similar fashion, and a drain is used to reduce the risk of postoperative seroma formation.

If shortening is not possible, 2 options are available. The first is to shorten to the next higher level of amputation, an option that, for obvious reasons, many amputees do not like. The second option is a free tissue transfer to gain soft tissue over the stump. This operation is technically difficult and requires a surgeon with expertise in microvascular transfers.

Three types of flaps are available for transfer: fasciocutaneous flaps, musculocutaneous flaps, and muscle-only flaps. The flap must be tailored to the individual stump, but in most cases the authors prefer musculocutaneous flap. The authors have also experienced slightly higher rates of flap loss and complications in flaps that cross the knee joint. Recovery time to prosthetic wearing may also be prolonged depending on how long it takes for the flap to completely heal. For these reasons, patients should be carefully selected for these procedures and be well educated on the process.

The other indication for revision of a stump is to attempt to reduce pain while wearing a prosthesis. Patients for this type of revision must be carefully selected. The first challenge is to properly diagnose the pain generator, most often a painful neuroma. These patients complain of electrical pain or burning-type pain that limits prosthetic wear and is relieved by removing the prosthesis. Patients with below-knee amputations with electrical pain that radiates to the bottom of the foot likely have tibial nerve pain, and those with pain to the top if the foot typically have peroneal nerve pain.

A Tinel sign over the nerve can usually be elicited. A local anesthetic injection or block can be helpful if it does relieve pain in the prosthesis. Lack of response is more difficult to interpret.

For patients with peroneal nerve pain, the authors typically resect the nerve over the fibular head and transpose it into a muscle belly of the hamstrings above the knee. A curvilinear incision is made over the fibular head, and dissection is carried down to the fascia under tourniquet control. The nerve is identified as it crosses below the fibular head from posterior to anterior. The nerve is injected with local anesthetic, typically marcaine, then transected. It is then dissected proximally as far as possible. A second incision is made above the knee and the dissection is connected under the skin bridge. The nerve is then brought out the superior incision. It is then rerouted into the muscle belly above the knee and sutured into the muscle. Many times the authors will cap the nerve with a nerve tube with one end sutured shut; however, the efficacy of this maneuver is somewhat controversial. A pain pump is then placed adjacent to the nerve end, and the wounds are closed after the tourniquet is let down and hemostasis is obtained.

The tibial nerve is more difficult to locate more proximally with a limited dissection, and the authors will often try to locate the neuroma at the level of the stump and cut it back.

Patients must understand preoperatively that immediate pain relief should not be expected and that pain levels with often increase temporarily after this type of surgery. Aggressive postoperative pain control is important.

Targeted Muscle Reinnervation

Targeted reinnervation is a new neural-machine interface that has been developed to help improve the function of electrically powered upper prosthetic limbs.[1] It is a surgical procedure that takes the nerves that once innervated the amputated limb and replants them in proximal muscle and skin sites. The sensory afferents of the redirected nerves reinnervate the skin overlying the transfer site, creating a sensory expression of the missing limb in the amputee's reinnervated skin. When these individuals are touched on this reinnervated skin they feel as though they are being touched on their missing limb. Targeted reinnervation takes nerves that once served the hand, a skin region of high functional importance, and redirects them to less functionally relevant skin areas adjacent to the amputation site. Using this procedure produces more muscle-signal sites that can be used to operate the electric prosthesis.

Osseous Integration (Direct Skeletal Attachment)

Osseointegrated implants for prosthetic suspension offer amputees an alternative to the traditional socket suspension, and are especially useful for transfemoral and transhumeral levels of amputation. Potential benefits include a natural transfer of loads directly to the skeleton via a percutaneous abutment that is placed into the residual bone.[2] This procedure can also offer relief of pain and discomfort of residual limb soft tissues by eliminating sockets. In addition, there is increased sensory feedback and improved function because forces are directly transmitted to the distal prosthetic components. Despite the benefits, the skin-implant interface remains a limitation, as it can serve as an entrance to the residual limb for bacterial infection. In addition, there have been instances of long bone fracture proximal to the abutment.

Bone Lengthening and Soft-Tissue Coverage

Cadaver bone can be used to lengthen an extremely short residual bony lever arm. This procedure provides a longer residual limb to power the prosthesis. Allograft

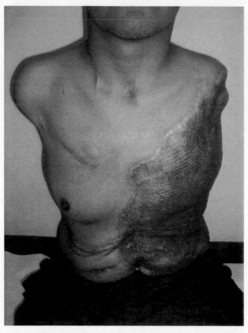

Fig. 3. A 26-year-old man with very short transhumeral arm amputation on the right side. Only the humeral head remains in the glenohumeral fossa on the right.

bone is attached using internal fixation to provide up to 15 cm of new bone length. Covering this new length with soft tissue becomes a challenge for the plastic surgeon, who may choose to rotate a full-thickness flap to cover the new bone. Split-thickness graft can be used to cover the portions of the new residual limb, which is less likely to have pressures placed on it by the socket of the prosthesis. This lengthening is especially useful in very short transhumeral and transradial residual limbs where a longer lever arm provides more useful prosthetic function (**Figs. 3–5**).

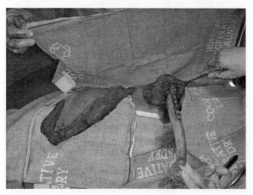

Fig. 4. The allograft has been attached to the residual humeral head using a metal plate. This new bone provides an additional 15 cm of length for the right residual arm.

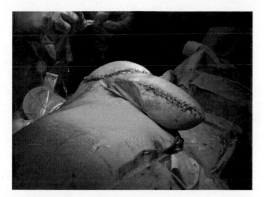

Fig. 5. The newly lengthened right arm is now covered with a pedicle latissimus dorsi flap that has been brought through the axilla to cover the allograft bone, providing full-thickness skin and muscle over the end of the now lengthened residual arm.

REFERENCES

1. Kuiken TA, Li G, Lock BA, et al. Targeted muscle reinnervation for real-time myoelectric control of multifunction artificial arms. JAMA 2009;301(6):619–28. http://dx.doi.org/10.1001/jama.2009.116.
2. Nebergall A, Bragdon C, Antonellis A, et al. Stable fixation of an osseointegrated implant system for above-the-knee amputees: Titel RSA and radiographic evaluation of migration and bone remodeling in 55 cases. Acta Orthop 2012;83(2):121–8. http://dx.doi.org/10.3109/17453674.2012.678799.

SELECTED READINGS

Barnes RW, Cox B. Amputations an illustrated manual. Philadelphia: Hanley&Belfus, Inc; 2000.
Bennett JB, Alexander CB. Amputation levels and surgical techniques, Chapter 2. In: Meier RH, Atkins DJ, editors. Functional restoration of adults and children with upper extremity amputation. New York: Demos; 2004. p. 9–22.
Bowker JH. Surgical management, Chapter 38. In: Smith DG, Michael JW, Bowker JH, editors. Atlas of amputation and limb deficiencies surgical, prosthetic and rehabilitation principles. 3rd edition. American Academy of Orthopaedic Surgery; 2004. p. 481–502.
Gottschalk F. Transfemoral amputation: surgical management, Chapter 42. In: Smith DG, Michael JW, Bowker JH, editors. Atlas of amputation and limb deficiencies surgical, prosthetic and rehabilitation principles. 3rd edition. American Academy of Orthopaedic Surgery; 2004. p. 533–40.
Shenaq SM, Grantcharova E. Upper extremity amputation revision and reconstruction, Chapter 4. In: Meier RH, Atkins DJ, editors. Functional restoration of adults and children with upper extremity amputation. New York: Demos; 2004. p. 35–42.
Smith DG. General principles of amputation surgery, Chapter 2. In: Smith DG, Michael JW, Bowker JH, editors. Atlas of amputation and limb deficiencies surgical, prosthetic and rehabilitation principles. 3rd edition. American Academy of Orthopaedic Surgery; 2004. p. 21–30.
Wilkins RM, Brown WC. Upper extremity salvage and reconstruction for trauma and tumors, Chapter 3. In: Meier RH, Atkins DJ, editors. Functional restoration of adults and children with upper extremity amputation. New York: Demos; 2004. p. 23–34.

Pain Issues and Treatment of the Person with an Amputation

Heikki Uustal, MD[a,b], Robert H. Meier III, MD[c,*]

KEYWORDS

- Pain issues • Amputation • Residual limb pain • Pain treatment algorithm
- Phantom limb pain

KEY POINTS

- The clinician must specifically define what patients with amputations mean when they relate that they have pain.
- The most common causative factor for residual limb pain is with the prosthetic fit.
- Standard pain medications can be useful in the acute postoperative period to control the postsurgical pain.
- The use of a pain treatment algorithm for the person with an amputation who is experiencing pain can provide a rational guide for the progression of treatment options.

Most people with amputations should not experience pain that interferes with their quality of life or requires regular medication more than 6 months following the amputation surgery.[1–13] In fact, most people with amputations do not experience significant pain more than 3 months following the amputation.

However, the clinician must specifically define what patients with amputations mean when they relate that they have pain. The pain must be carefully differentiated to treat it properly. By far, most problematic pain that is present more than 6 months after the amputation is related to a poorly fitting prosthesis and should be properly labeled as residual limb pain. This practice gets the treating physician to differentiate between nociceptive versus neuropathic pain. The most commonly used treatments can fit into 5 general categories: (1) medications, (2) prosthetic changes, (3) psychosocial treatments, (4) noninvasive therapies (ie, physical therapy, pain modalities), and (5) surgery.

Most people with acquired amputations experience phantom limb pain, at least in the acute postoperative period. This pain is carefully defined as pain that is present in the part of the limb that has been removed and not in the tissues of the limb that is remaining. Most often, this pain subsides but may be present for a split second

a JFK-Johnson Rehab Institute, 65 James Street, Edison, NJ 08820, USA; b Physical Medicine and Rehabilitation, Rutgers-Robert Wood Johnson Medical School, 675 Hoes Lane, Piscataway, NJ 08854, USA; c Amputee Services of America, 1601 East 19th Avenue, Suite 3200, Denver, CO 80218, USA
* Corresponding author.
E-mail address: skipdoc3@gmail.com

Phys Med Rehabil Clin N Am 25 (2014) 45–52
http://dx.doi.org/10.1016/j.pmr.2013.09.008
1047-9651/14/$ – see front matter © 2014 Elsevier Inc. All rights reserved.

on occasion throughout the life of people with amputations. Usually, however, it significantly decreases and does not require treatment beyond 3 months after the amputation surgery. It is also important that the phenomenon of phantom sensation be differentiated from phantom pain. Most people with acquired amputations will experience some phantom sensation throughout their lives. However, the amount of phantom sensation will usually diminish over time. This experience is described as feeling that the amputated portion of the limb is still present. With time, the distal end of the limb (hand or foot) will move closer to the end of the residual limb, which is called *telescoping*. It is important to explain this experience to the patients with new amputations so they better understand that it is a real phenomenon that is to be expected and that will change over time.

Residual limb pain is defined as pain that is present in some part of the limb that remains following the amputation. There are a variety of potential causes of this type of pain, and these require a careful history and investigation in order to provide a treatment approach that is likely to decrease the pain and not result in chronic medication use or opiate addiction.

One of the presently confounding things in pain treatment are the number of medications and modalities that are available for use to try to diminish the pain experience. Sherman wrote about many of these modalities in the 1970s and 1980s. Most of these treatments are in use today, but now we have many more treatment options to try. One of the problems in treatment is the physicians themselves. We now have a subspecialty in pain management, and many of these physicians do not have extensive knowledge in musculoskeletal anatomy, kinesiology, proper prosthetic fitting techniques, or the mechanics of prosthetic function or gait analysis. All of these areas enter into the proper assessment and treatment of people with amputations who have pain. Another issue in pain treatment is the need for careful follow-up and treatment coordination. There is a tendency to shotgun treatment rather than take time to carefully try one modality before adding another treatment or several treatments at a time. Thus, the pain treatment algorithm for the person with an amputation has been developed (**Figs. 1** and **2**).

In addition to specific treatment modalities, there are several lifestyle changes that will assist to diminish the pain experience. These changes can be more difficult to achieve than simply providing a medication or a transcutaneous electrical stimulation (TENS) unit. These changes include the following: (1) cessation of smoking, (2) decrease in stress, (3) decrease in depression, (4) control of edema, (5) distraction from the pain, and (6) increasing activity level.

RESIDUAL LIMB PAIN

The most common causative factor for residual limb pain is with the prosthetic fit. In an amputation with prosthetic restoration, pressures are put on tissues of the remaining leg or arm that were not designed to be pressure bearing. Most sockets require an intimate fit to provide maximum function and provide pressure points that can often be uncomfortable or painful. For the people with transtibial leg amputations, these points are often the fibular head or the distal anterior kick point. In people with transfemoral amputations, this point is usually the distal lateral area where the distal femur comes in contact with the lateral socket wall. This point of contact is essential for keeping the pelvis as level as possible during the stance phase of the above-knee prosthesis. In the arm prostheses, it is often the distal ends of the radius and ulna for people with transradial amputations and the distal anterior end of the humerus for people with transhumeral amputations.

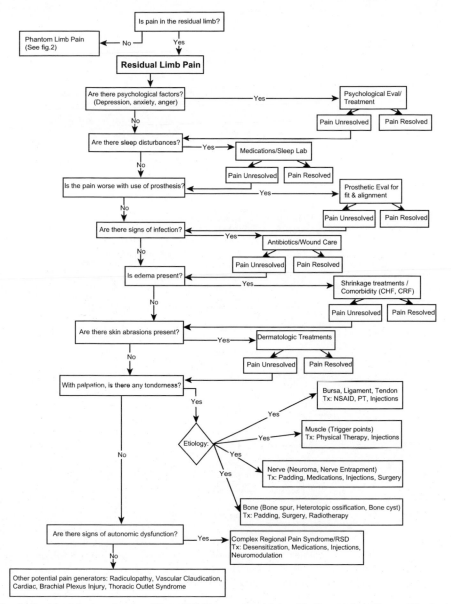

Fig. 1. Residual limb pain algorithm. NSAID, nonsteroidal antiinflammatory drugs; PT, physical therapy. (*From* Hompland S. Pain management for upper extremity amputation. In: Meier RH, Atkins DJ, editors. Functional restoration of adults and children with upper extremity amputation. New York: Demos, 2004; with permission.)

Residual limb pain may be caused when the socket exerts excess pressure on the residual limb soft tissues, especially on nerves or a neuroma that has formed at the cut end of a peripheral nerve.

In some cases, residual limb pain is a result of the underlying bone changes that could be bony overgrowth from the margins of the cut bone or the development of

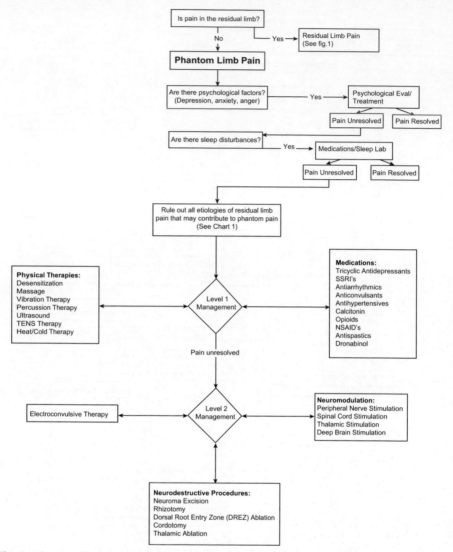

Fig. 2. Phantom limb pain algorithm. (*From* Hompland S. Pain management for upper extremity amputation. In: Meier RH, Atkins DJ, editors. Functional restoration of adults and children with upper extremity amputation. New York: Demos, 2004; with permission.)

heterotopic bone within the soft tissues of the residual limb. These painful bone growths may require surgical removal.

An additional consideration for pain generation in the person with an amputation should be musculoskeletal imbalance. All people with amputations have an alteration in their usual body mechanics. Often this results in a musculoskeletal imbalance that is often seen in a change in their posture. It is common that myofascial pain becomes a secondary source of pain in the affected extremity or the contralateral extremity.

Last but not least as a cause for residual limb pain is the presence of the pathophysiology that caused the amputation. Is there a peripheral neuropathy that is causing the pain? Was there a nerve insult during the traction injury that led to the amputation? Is there claudication because of the original dysvascular disease that caused the amputation? Has the tumor that required the amputation returned? Is infection brewing within the bone or soft tissues, which is causing the residual limb pain?

PHANTOM LIMB PAIN

Phantom limb pain is usually present for a few weeks following the amputation and subsides over time, with an occasional occurrence that is usually over in an instant. Phantom limb pain should not require opiates or synthetic opiate medication for more than 3 months and often less. For whatever reason, phantom pain seems to be more problematic in people with arm amputations than in people with leg amputations. With prolonged (greater than 6 months) phantom pain that is severe, the quality of life can be greatly reduced and narcotic addiction or medication tolerance is often present.

GENERALIZED TREATMENT MODALITIES THAT SHOULD ALWAYS BE USED

The following list contains modalities that should always be used when phantom pain is present and causing any distress for people with amputations:

1. Control edema present in the stump
2. Establish a restful sleep pattern (at least 6 hours of uninterrupted sleep a night)
3. Decrease anxiety
4. Decrease stress
5. Restore the locus of control of their life to the person with the amputation
6. Restore meaningful function
7. Use desensitization techniques for the residual limb
8. Decrease depression
9. Cessation of smoking

Cessation of smoking is a must if pain control is a continuing problem and there is any hope of decreasing the phantom pain.

RESIDUAL LIMB EVALUATION FOR PAIN

Prosthetic fit has already been mentioned as a common cause for residual limb pain. The physician evaluating the person for pain must assess the fit of the prosthetic socket, and this assessment may also require input from the prosthetist who has fabricated the prosthesis. Prosthetic suspension may also contribute to the pain by causing shear or drag on the soft tissues during prosthetic wearing and function.

If people with amputations have a diabetic neuropathy or have had an extremity traction injury, there may be neuropathic pain present. Often pain in the residual limb is attributed to the presence of a neuroma. As is known, all amputations result in neuroma formation, but only a few of these lead to problematic pain. If on palpation, a neuroma is felt and pressure on that neuroma reproduces the pain experience, then it is likely the source of the pain. On occasion, magnetic resonance imaging of the residual limb is helpful is visualizing the presence, size, and location of a problematic neuroma.

Even if a neuroma is present, if the cause of the amputation was dysvascular disease, claudication in the limb should be considered as a cause of residual limb pain. The vascular supply to the remaining limb should be assessed.

Control of edema in the amputated limb is essential, especially when the prosthesis is not being worn. Edema in itself may result in a painful situation. Residual limb volume measurements may be necessary in order to assess the amount of edema that is forming in the limb.

Assessment for bony prominences or new bone formation is best accomplished with careful palpation of the bone and soft tissues of the residual limb. In addition, a plain film may help establish the contours of the bony edges. On occasion, the prominence of bony edges is related to whether a myoplastic closure was performed or that the myoplastic closure has come apart. In this situation, the pain may be produced when the bony edges are immediately under the skin with no other soft tissue padding to be protective during prosthetic wearing.

MEDICATIONS

Standard pain medications can be useful in the acute postoperative period to control the postsurgical pain. However, if phantom pain enters the pain picture, then pregabalin seems to provide better results in alleviating the phantom pain than gabapentin does. In addition, whichever of these medications is used for treating phantom pain, their dosages should be increased every 2 weeks until there is good pain relief or toxicity is present. Because there is a temptation to provide pain relief as quickly as possible, often many medications are thrown at the problem. Multiple medication use makes it difficult to know which, if any, of the medications in use might be providing the most effective pain relief. It is more effective if one pain treatment method is changed at a time to be able to discern which treatment is most efficacious.

There are several alternative medications that are in use today. Because the author is in a state where the use of marijuana is considered legal within the state, reports from patients indicate that, for some, marijuana is the only substance that provides adequate pain relief. A way to test this using a legal substance is to try dronabinol to see if it provides pain relief compared with the other medications that have been used.

THERAPEUTIC MODALITIES

Several noninvasive modalities can be tried to see what effect they might have to decrease the pain. These modalities need to be applied by an experienced therapist and used in a rationale manner for an appropriate period of time before they are deemed helpful or not. These modalities include but are not limited to the following:

1. Desensitization techniques
2. Massage, both scar and soft tissue
3. Edema control
4. Ultrasound
5. TENS
6. Exercise
7. Hot/cold contrast
8. Interferential current
9. Mirror therapy

MISCELLANEOUS PAIN TREATMENT MODALITIES

Several other modalities for pain treatment have come into and gone out of vogue. If they are to be used, they need to be provided by a skilled therapist. These modalities include the following:

1. Acupuncture
2. Magnets
3. Farabloc (Farabloc Development Corp, Coquitlam, BC)
4. Biofeedback
5. Electromagnetic stimulation
6. Kinesiotherapy
7. Eye Movement Desensitization and Reprocessing (see article by Belon and Vigoda, elsewhere in this issue)

PSYCHOLOGIC FACTORS THAT INFLUENCE THE PAIN EXPERIENCE

The relationship between the pain experience and the emotional well-being of patients with amputations cannot be overemphasized. To treat one without understanding the influence of the other is foolhardy and shortsighted. To divorce these issues is only treating a part of patients and does not provide comprehensive medical care. There are many emotional challenges for patients with amputations, especially in the early postamputation phase. The issues to be considered should include the following: (1) loss of life control, (2) anxiety, (3) changes in body image, (4) changes in functional abilities, (5) depression, (6) sleep disturbance, (7) eating disturbance, and (8) nightmares (daymares, flashbacks) and posttraumatic stress disorder. These issues and their treatment are discussed in the article by Belon and Vigoda, elsewhere in this issue.

INVASIVE TECHNIQUES FOR PAIN TREATMENT

For some patients with amputation pain who have not found relief with more conservative pain treatments, a more invasive form of management may be appropriate. The most simple of these is represented by an injection in the area of a neuroma. Often this technique uses a local anesthetic that may be combined with an injectable steroid medication. In some cases, a sympathetic block or blocks are tried to see if there is a significant sympathetic contribution to the pain.

Revision of the residual limb with resection of a neuroma can also be successful, but the neuroma may also return. Other nerve surgery may use peripheral nerve stimulation for pain relief. In some cases, a trial of spinal stimulation is warranted, and consideration for the implantation of a permanent spinal cord stimulator is appropriate.

Central nervous system surgery has been attempted in the past but without consistent success. The techniques include a dorsal root entry zone procedure or brain stimulation.

USE OF A PAIN TREATMENT ALGORITHM FOR THE PERSON WITH AN AMPUTATION WITH PROBLEMATIC PAIN

The use of a pain treatment algorithm for a person with an amputation who is experiencing pain can provide a rational guide for the progression of treatment options. Although the differentiation of phantom limb pain from residual limb pain has been presented, the 2 pain phenomena may occur simultaneously. However, the treatment of one type of amputation pain is usually quite different than the other treatment options. The algorithm suggested here does try to separate these 2 differing types of pain and the treatment options available. In both algorithms, the least invasive and less complex treatments are offered first, progressing through the more complex and invasive options.

If the pain-treating physician is 4 months into using these algorithms without signs of pain relief, then another specialist may need to provide some input to the treatment options, especially if a lot of narcotic or synthetic narcotic is still required. By this time, most people with amputations will have had a significant decrease in their post-amputation pain and not require regular medication or the stronger pain medications. Dependency can be a real issue at this time; other factors may be driving the need for medication, not just the presence of pain.

REFERENCES

1. Hompland S. Pain management for upper extremity amputation. Chaper 9. In: Meier RH, Atkins DJ, editors. Functional restoration of adults and children with upper extremity amputation. New York: Demos; 2004. p. 89–112.
2. Sherman RA, Sherman CJ, Gall NG. A survey of current phantom limb treatment in the United States. Pain 1980;8:85–99.
3. Mitchell SW. Injuries of nerves and their consequences. Philadelphia: J.B. Lippincott; 1872.
4. Sherman RA, Sherman CJ. A comparison of phantom sensations among amputees whose amputations were of civilian and military origins. Pain 1985;21:91.
5. Melzack R. Phantom limb pain: implications for treatment of pathologic pain. Anesthesiology 1971;35:409–19.
6. Sherman RA, Gall N, Gormly J. Treatment of limb pain with muscular relaxation training to disrupt the pain-anxiety-tension cycle. Pain 1979;6:47.
7. Dworkin RH. Which individuals with acute pain are most likely to develop a chronic pain syndrome? Pain Forum 1997;6:127–36.
8. Fordyce WE. Behavioral methods for chronic pain and illness. St Louis (MO): Mosby-Year Book; 1976.
9. Jensen MP, Turner JA, Romano JM, et al. Relationship of pain-specific beliefs to chronic pain adjustment. Pain 1994;57:301–9.
10. Ehde DM, Czernicki JM, Smith DG. Chronic phantom sensations, phantom pain, residual limb pain and other regional pain after lower limb amputation. Arch Phys Med Rehabil 2000;81:1039–44.
11. Jensen TS, Krebs B, Nielsen J, et al. Immediate and long-term phantom limb pain in amputees: incidence, clinical characteristics and relationship to pre-amputation limb pain. Pain 1985;21:267–78.
12. Czerniecki JM, Ehde DM. Pain after lower extremity amputation. Crit Rev Phys Med Rehabil 2003;15:309–32.
13. Huse E, Larbig W, Flor H, et al. The effect of opioids on phantom limb pain and cortical reorganization. Pain 2001;90:47–55.

Emotional Adaptation to Limb Loss

Howard P. Belon, PhD*, Diane F. Vigoda, LCSW, CCM

KEYWORDS

• Emotional responses • Grieving • Grief resolution • Coping strategies

KEY POINTS

- Individuals experience multiple changes as a result of amputation. These changes not only are physical in nature (body image and functional abilities) but also may include psychological, financial, and comfort changes across the spectrum of an individual's life.
- It is important to assess the emotional responses that an individual may experience postsurgery and throughout the rehabilitation process. Grieving is a natural and normal emotional response that all amputees experience postamputation. Grief resolution is one of the primary areas of focus in counseling amputees.
- The development of effective coping strategies aids in the physical and emotional functional well-being of an amputee. Some of the more common strategies include relaxation training, use of exercise, maintaining a balanced diet, identifying and addressing negative self-talk, pacing, and eye movement desensitization and reprocessing (EMDR), frequently used to treat posttraumatic stress syndromes.
- In the effective treatment of individuals with amputation, it is imperative to assess the emotional adjustments of individuals to change. This article examines various factors and strategies used in the adaptation and recovery from amputation.

When treating amputees, it is essential that medical professionals recognize not only the physical changes that amputation represents but also a series of other social, emotional, psychological, and economic issues that have an impact on a patient's rehabilitation.

CHANGES IMPOSED BY AMPUTATION

There are several reasons for loss of limb, or amputation. Amputation may be congenital or due to tumor, trauma, disease, and/or infection. It may occur without any notice,

Funding Sources: None.
Conflict of Interest: None.
Amputee Services of America, 1601 East 19th Avenue, Suite #5100, Denver, CO 80218, USA
* Corresponding author.
E-mail address: drhbelon@gmail.com

immediately after an accident. It may be a necessary part of medical treatment or performed to increase functionality. Regardless of the cause, amputation imposes several changes. Just as individuals are unique, so are their responses to and experiences resulting from amputation: physical changes as well as emotional and psychological. Treatment must address and involve all three of these areas in order to obtain a positive outcome.

Changes in Body Image

Significant body image changes occur. Except for cases of congenital anomaly, humans are born with two arms and two legs. Looking at a mirror, individuals are used to seeing themselves in a certain way; clothes fit in a familiar manner; there is symmetry and balance to the human body. Someone who experiences amputation may feel incomplete, no longer whole. For some, loss of any body part, even a finger or toe, may be perceived as a gross disfigurement. Individuals may no longer feel attractive by societal standards.

Changes in Functional Abilities

Young children learn to roll over, crawl, stand, and walk. They learn to grasp objects and use their arms and hands for everyday activities. Using limbs and digits becomes second nature. They do not analyze how to break down muscle movement in order to complete everyday tasks. All of this changes postamputation. Necessary adaptations include learning to use muscles and limbs/digits in different manners, building up different muscles, using adaptive equipment and/or modifications, and using prostheses or learning new techniques to complete activities. Additional time is required, at least initially, to complete tasks. Adjusting is a frustrating process that requires assistance (therapists, aides, and family members) immediately after amputation. With time, practice, and the development of new techniques to accomplish various tasks, the ease of completing them should rapidly increase. It is also important for amputees to confront that there may be some tasks they never will be able to complete.

Changes in Finances

Amputation frequently has an impact on individual and family finances. If injured at work, individuals may receive long-term and short-term disability payments, usually a percentage of their previous income. Additionally, many find they are unable to work in their established field or even find employment, especially in an already tight job market.

Medical insurance coverage is another area that can have an impact on finances negatively. Certain insurance policies have yearly deductibles in addition to copayments for services, such as hospitalization, physician care, medical procedures, medications, equipment, and follow-up therapy, many of which frequently require preauthorization. Care and services may be delayed or denied by an insurance company, causing additional patient stress and frustration.

Medicare is a federal program that provides medical insurance to those who are 65 years of age and older or who are deemed disabled. To qualify, an individual (or spouse) must have worked at least 30 quarterly hours and paid into the Medicare system. To qualify for Medicare before age 65, someone must be deemed disabled and qualify for Social Security disability income (SSDI). The process to become eligible for SSDI benefits is long, tedious, and frustrating. It is not uncommon for an individual to be denied SSDI benefits 2 or 3 times, and legal assistance may be required to appeal eligibility denials. Once approved for SSDI benefits, there is a 2-year waiting period (from the date of eligibility determination), before Medicare benefits become active. Once approved for SSDI and Medicare, issues of copayments for services remain. In the meantime, there may be little household income, and patients may find themselves without insurance.

For those without medical insurance or who are underinsured, the cost of amputation and related services can create insurmountable debt. Those without insurance may qualify for state-assisted medical care (Medicaid), but there frequently are wait lists for these programs. Just as with most insurance programs, Medicaid also requires copayments for services.

The overall consequences associated with changes in income resulting from amputation can be devastating. With a loss of income, individuals prioritize their monthly bills. They may have to forgo paying for medications to cover rent/mortgage. If they cannot pay the rent/mortgage, they need to find affordable housing and move. Some cash out retirement/savings accounts, stocks/bonds, and their children's college funds to pay the mounting medical bills; many file for bankruptcy.

Changes in Comfort

There are many emotional and physical changes associated with adaptation to amputation. While trying to adapt to their situation, it is common for amputees to isolate themselves from family and friends. Their interactions with others may become stilted or awkward as both sides try to muddle through the situation and interact as if there are no changes. As a result of financial changes, such as those discussed previously, amputees may find that they have to change their lifestyle, because they are financially unable to participate in various activities (eg, going out to dinner or the movies).

Some experience pain after amputation, which may be physical and/or neuropathic in nature. To alleviate pain, medications may be prescribed. Medications may help resolve pain but also carry with them side effects that may affect an individual's comfort levels (personality changes from medications, changes in bowel/bladder, sexual functioning, and so forth).

When people experience physical, emotional, and psychological changes, changes occur to their homeostatic environments; they frequently experience anxiety, depression, or a mix of both emotions. These emotional responses are discussed further.

EMOTIONAL REACTIONS TO LIMB LOSS

The loss of a limb is similar to other major losses in life, especially what is near and dear. In its intensity and degree of impact, the loss of a limb probably comes closest, however, to the experience most encounter when losing a loved one. Just as it is natural to grieve the death of someone loved, amputees must grieve the loss of their limb, body integrity, and the people they used to be. Moreover, patients feel a loss of control over the limb loss process and their medical care. The initial period after amputation can be stressful, during which emotions can be raw and intense and feel out of control. Many amputees are confused by these emotions and wonder if they are "going crazy." It is best to warn new amputees of this possibility and let them know that grieving is a normal and natural process. They also should be encouraged to express and communicate their feelings to others, without trying to block or impede them. This likely makes it easier for them to accept and adapt to their amputation.

Kübler-Ross[1] was the first to identify and delineate the stages or steps that are gone through emotionally when faced with impending death or that of a loved one. She believed that each stage is proceeded through sequentially until reaching the final stage of acceptance. **Fig. 1** shows how she viewed individuals progressing through the stages of loss.

Dr. Kubler-Ross made a tremendous contribution to the field by acknowledging the importance of grieving and acceptance around death and dying. Her sequential model is probably too rigid to apply to the emotional experiences amputees face. Rather than proceeding steadily through a series of prescribed stages toward the final stage of acceptance, observations have shown that amputees experience a range of emotional reactions that can change from one moment to the next. Emotions can go back and forth along the continuum toward acceptance. Sometimes individuals may become stuck in a particular stage and remain there for some time. Not everyone experiences all of the stages. **Fig. 2** shows our view of how the grief process occurs.

Through this dynamic process, an adaptation to amputation eventually emerges. The important message to convey to amputees is that is natural to experience a wide variety of emotions, especially after a traumatic amputation. Those in the position to choose amputation may begin the grieving process from the moment they begin to contemplate it or as soon as they make their decision to have it. Others, like their peers who lost their limbs through trauma, wait until after amputation to process their feelings when faced with reality.

Many amputees find talking to a counselor beneficial in dealing with the grief and adjustments they face after an amputation. A Turkish proverb states, "He that conceals his grief finds no remedy for it." This is why the authors encourage most of amputee patients to participate in individual counseling, group counseling, or both. Sharing and expressing their feelings to someone who is objective and removed from their normal social support network may ease the burden shouldered by family and friends who, like amputees, often experience distress and probably

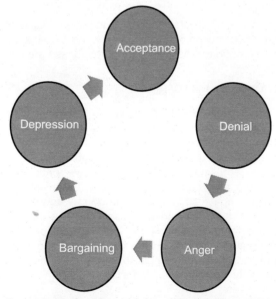

Fig. 1. The Kübler-Ross stages of coping with loss. (*Adapted from* Kübler-Ross E. On death and dying. New York: Macmillan; 1969.)

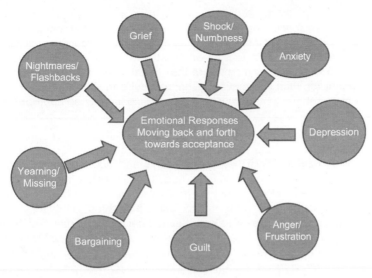

Fig. 2. The grief process.

are in the throes of their own grief process. However much they want to help, family and friends are not trained professionals and may not know how to respond to an amputee's particular emotional needs. A counselor can provide support, teach a variety of coping skills, and identify psychological obstacles that may be getting in the way.

Some of the typical emotional reactions amputees experience are discussed.

Shock and Disbelief

Typically, most amputees experience shock and disbelief after hearing they need an amputation or after amputation surgery itself. During this stage, most people find themselves confused, in disbelief, and unable to comprehend the magnitude and significance of what the amputation means for their lives from this point forward. It is common to feel dazed, as if in a dream or a nightmare. During this time, individuals may feel emotionally numb or as if they are just going through the motions. Others may find themselves tearful or even sobbing. Some experience sleeping problems, appetite loss, or loss of concentration or the ability to make even simple decisions. Those who become stuck in this stage usually have difficulty dealing with the hurdles typically encountered during rehabilitation due to their constant state of disbelief and disorientation, even over minor or trivial obstacles.

Denial

If shock and disbelief help block out the magnitude of what has happened and insulate amputees from overwhelming emotional pain, denial allows them to manage reality by not thinking about it or by minimizing the amputation's impact on their lives. Patients in this stage may act as if the amputation is no big deal and believe that once they receive their prosthesis they will be able to function as they did before. In the extreme, patients may take on a Pollyanna attitude, that everything is good. They may appear overly cheerful and positive. Indeed, such individuals may be viewed as model patients because they are so positive. Yet the reason they respond this way is to deny or avoid facing the negative aspects of their disability. It is important that medical caregivers monitor patients in denial as closely as they do those who are more expressive of their emotions; delayed grief reactions may occur at any time. Patients may eventually verbalize their concerns to one member of their health care team and not the others, so it is important for such information to be conveyed to the other team members when it occurs. A referral to a mental health professional may be appropriate at this time.

Anger

As reality begins to sink in, denial may turn into anger and rage. It is common to repeatedly ask, "Why me?" Additional questions or self-statements often follow, such as, "This isn't fair!" "How can this happen to me?" and "Who is to blame?" Anger can be experienced in several different forms, including frustration, annoyance, and irritation. Those who formerly were slow to lose their temper suddenly may find themselves with little patience and a short fuse. This stage is most pronounced for people who think that their amputations were a result of other people's errors, neglect, or ineptitude. They resent those responsible for their limb loss. Others who have undergone an amputation after illness or disease may feel bitter that life is unfair or unjust to allow cancer or diabetes to take their limb. Sometimes people blame God for their problems; often they blame themselves, especially if they believe they had a part in causing the amputation to happen.

Our society is very conflicted about anger. Many individuals are raised or socialized to believe that having or expressing anger is bad and they need to avoid it at all costs, usually by keeping it inside. Repressing anger, however, may exact a heavy price; anger that is not expressed outwardly can turn inward and be channeled physically, causing stomach ulcers, pain, and other physical ailments. The repression of feelings can amplify residual limb pain or phantom pain. Moreover, amputees who avoid expressing their anger may become more irritable and easily strike out or snap at those closest to them, such as family members, friends, caregivers, or medical staff. Those who remain stuck in this stage tend to be indiscriminant when it comes to directing their anger toward others.

Depression

With depression, the question remains, "Why me?" But with depression, rather than feeling angry toward their circumstances, patients feel sorry for themselves. Freud[2] once defined depression as "anger turned inward." These patients typically feel victimized, hopeless, and helpless. Depression usually leads to fatigue, apathy, and loss of interest or pleasure in activities that used to be enjoyable. It is often difficult to concentrate and find the energy to do even the littlest things. Some may feel overly sad, melancholy, and tearful; others may feel detached and emotionally numb.

The following symptoms are consistent in many individuals diagnosed as depressed[3]:

1. Depressed mood most of the day nearly every day
2. Markedly diminished interest or pleasure in all or almost all activities most of the day
3. Significant weight loss or weight gain
4. Insomnia or hypersomnia nearly every day
5. Psychomotor agitation or retardation nearly every day

6. Fatigue or loss of energy nearly every day
7. Feelings of worthlessness or excessive or inappropriate guilt
8. Diminished ability to think or concentrate
9. Recurrent thoughts of death or suicidal ideation or a suicide attempt

The physical components of depression may be confusing. Amputees may interpret their symptoms of lethargy and fatigue as signs of their worsening physical health (eg, increased pain complaints). This may prompt pessimism about the future, which is likely to feed right back into their depression. As more depressed is felt, pain can increase and vice versa. This can lead to a vicious pain-depression cycle. Although the type of depression in this stage is usually situational, if an amputee also has a biologic depression (ie, a depressive predisposition that is inherited), the depression may become even more severe and prolonged.

Anxiety

Amputees may become nervous, anxious, or even panicked about their future life as an amputee. They may wonder, "What do I do now?" Some worry that their lives are over or that they have no future. The fear of the unknown is frightening. Some worry about rational threats or dangers the future may bring. Those who undergo amputation as a result of developing cancer in a limb may wonder if all the cancer was removed or their cancer will return in the future. They may catastrophize or worry about the worst things happening to them, such as eventually dying from cancer. Others fear they may not be able to work again, their finances will crumble, and their marriages will dissolve. Such worry can generate physical tension, causing shakiness, insomnia, panic attacks, and increased pain.

Those whose amputations were the result of traumatic events, such as car or work-related accidents or combat, may experience symptoms associated with anxiety and trauma. They may have nightmares or flashbacks of the trauma, often unpredictably. This is normal because it is the mind's way of working through, or digesting, the trauma. Nightmares often occur because there is less control of thoughts and feelings while asleep; it is easier for the traumatic experiences and memories to leak into dreams. When anxiety and trauma become severe, posttraumatic stress disorder (PTSD) may develop. Symptoms of PTSD include[3]

Intrusive memories
- Flashbacks, or reliving the traumatic event for minutes or even days at a time
- Upsetting dreams about the traumatic event
Avoidance and emotional numbing
- Trying to avoid thinking or talking about the traumatic event
- Feeling emotionally numb
- Avoiding activities previously enjoyed
- Hopelessness about the future
- Memory problems
- Trouble concentrating
- Difficulty maintaining close relationships
Anxiety and increased emotional arousal
- Irritability or anger
- Overwhelming guilt or shame
- Self-destructive behavior, such as drinking too much
- Trouble sleeping
- Being easily startled or frightened
- Hallucinations, such as hearing or seeing things that are not there

Guilt

Guilt is an affective state in which people experience conflict at having done some-thing that they believe they should not have done or, conversely, not having done something they believe they should have done. It gives rise to a feeling that does not go away easily, driven by conscience. Amputees may feel guilt and regret for what they perceive as their fault for causing their amputation. They may feel respon-sible for having caused the accident that took their limb or they may blame themselves for not taking care of themselves by eating too much, not exercising enough, working too hard, smoking, and so forth.

Guilt also may come from feeling bad about the losses and changes that occur after amputation. For example, individuals who used to be a primary breadwinner in the family may feel guilt because they no longer are able to support their family financially. They are heartbroken when watching their spouses go off to work while they stay home feeling helpless and useless, without much structure or direction in their lives. For many men, work often defines their character or sense of identity. When their work is stripped away, they may experience a major blow to their ego, which can be devastating to their self-esteem and self-worth. The hopes and dreams they may have had for themselves and their families no longer seem possible, and they may feel guilty for letting everybody down.

Bargaining

Bargaining may occur prior to loss as well as afterward. When faced with a life-threatening choice of either dying or losing a limb, most people opt to avoid death and choose amputation. Many cancer and diabetic patients make this choice every day. Others may not be faced with such clear-cut, life-and-death decisions. Some might choose amputation as a way to avoid pain or maintain function. In their minds, they are striking a bargain, "If I do this difficult thing, something good will come out of it." In other words, "If I give up my limb, I won't have to worry about dying." Bargaining is a way of trying to gain control over an unfortunate situation—an attempt to interject logic and rationality into a situation that may seem perplexing, uncertain, and fright-ening. Some negotiate with a higher power, someone or something they perceive as having control over the situation. They may make promises to God in return for their amputation working out successfully and their lives being spared. Bargaining may lead to an easier acceptance of amputation because patients who have survived, and not died, may be better positioned to accept the terms of their grand bargain, namely accepting their amputee status.

Yearning

In a recent study, Zhang and colleagues[4] found that most people's primary negative feeling after a loss was not sadness or anger, as previously thought, but yearning. In-dividuals often deeply miss a loved one who has died, wishing they still were with them. Individuals may hold out hope, despite knowing intellectually that they are not coming back. Many find reassurance in their faith that someday, in the afterlife, they will meet their loved ones again. Prigerson[5] says, "Grief is really about yearning and not sadness... That sense of heartache. It's been called pangs of grief." In a similar manner, yearning to have back a limb is common after amputation. A few patients have expressed belief that their limbs will grow back. Although technical features of prosthetics and what they can do have come a long way in recent years, they are still not full replacements for limbs. Patients begin to realize this as soon as they receive their artificial limbs and become aware of their limitations.

Amputees may yearn for the old days when they had all their all their limbs intact. They also may yearn for the way things were when they had gainful employment, were earning an income, had their health, and were able to do activities without thinking about it. It is typical for amputees to miss their former carefree selves who did not take a long time to dress and care for themselves the way they do as amputees.

Acceptance

Although Kübler-Ross believed that attaining acceptance was the final stage of grief, Zhang and colleagues[4] found that acceptance was not the final stage but that it comes and goes throughout the grieving process. It was the most common feeling among those who were grieving and it often occurred early in the grieving process. For amputees, acceptance is often reflected in the adjustments, accommodations, and adaptations they begin to make from the moment they undergo amputation. One of the first adaptations required of leg amputees is using a wheelchair to get around while wearing a cast on the leg and then a removable cast (eg, clamshell). They may eventually switch to a walker and later use forearm crutches or a cane. Arm amputees, on the other hand, may have to learn how to use new eating utensils. Even prostheses require making adjustments in using muscles, coordination, and balance as well as the time and effort it takes to don and remove the prosthesis.

People are adaptable beings and have learned to adapt to some of the most inhospitable environments, including the frigid cold of Antarctica, the barren sand of the Sahara desert, and the weightless environs of outer space. Similarly, most amputees are able to go with the flow as they accept and deal with each step in the rehabilitation process. Through successful adaptation with each new step, amputees realize that they can go on with their lives if they are willing to be flexible and make accommodations to the way they previously did things. Consequently, they may start to experience more good days than bad ones. Anger and depression may subside, as amputees feel more confident about being able to move forward and realize they have a future. They begin to get back to participating in some of the pleasurable activities they used to do before amputation, albeit with adjustments, or learn new activities—such as skiing—while working around their physical limitations through the use of adaptable equipment, learning new skills, and applying new techniques. As amputees accept that they have to do things differently, they learn that their lives do not have to stop and that they can live their lives in a new but different way. As one amputee put it recently, "I accept my amputation, but I don't have to like it."

COPING STRATEGIES

Amputees can learn a variety of coping strategies for dealing with the psychological effects of their amputations. Most of these strategies are based on cognitive-behavior and mindfulness approaches. Because it takes practice to build skills, they are instructed to practice these strategies regularly but in moderation. Too little practice results in their forgetting to use the strategies; using them too much can lead to burnout and a tendency to quit. **Fig. 3** shows the need to find a balance for each intervention.

Just as a bicycle wheel's spokes must be balanced for it to turn smoothly, these skills are best used in a balanced manner. When the spokes are out of balance, the wheel is wobbly and moves inefficiently. The same can be said for people: when they do not use their coping skills in a balanced manner, their ability to handle stress is less effective and efficient. Individuals identify which areas they need to build up and

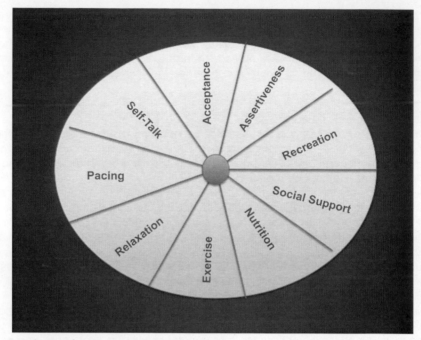

Fig. 3. Balance of amputee interventional skills.

are instructed to work on one intervention at a time until they are practicing all of these strategies on a routine basis.

Relaxation Training

One of the first skills taught is relaxation. Patients are offered a variety of techniques to release physical tension, manage anxiety, control pain, and destress themselves. This enables them to feel more empowered and centered with a greater sense of well-being. At first, they are introduced to the principles and method of diaphragmatic breathing, the deep breathing that is the foundation of all forms of relaxation. It is easy to do, portable, and takes little time; most patients find it enjoyable.

They are encouraged to follow the 3-in-1 rule: take 3 deep breaths once an hour. Of course, they can take more than 3 breaths at shorter intervals (eg, every one-half hour or every 15 minutes). Most are willing to do this, but because breathing is usually on automatic pilot, it is common for them to forget. Because people do not typically focus on breathing, and to help remind patients do so, they can create a cuing system that signals when it is time to stop and breathe deeply. Most people are able to set their watch or cell phone to chime every hour, reminding them to practice diaphragmatic breathing.

It is ironic that human beings spend so little time aware of their breathing processes, because they cannot live long without oxygen. People pay more attention to other bodily needs—eating, drinking, sleeping, or sex—than to breathing. It is recommended that patients set aside 20 to 30 minutes to practice the technique while lying down, when it is easier to watch the abdomen moving up and down. Patients can put a book on their belly to make it easier to watch the movement of their abdomen. Once they become tired of observing their breath, they might close their eyes and pay attention to the pleasant sensation of rhythmic breathing. In this way, they can get more fully in touch with their breathing and appreciate its importance for their body.

Other relaxation techniques that benefit amputees include visualization/guided imagery (eg, imagining taking a vacation in a safe, relaxing place), meditation, yoga, Tai Chi, biofeedback, and self-hypnosis. Listening to relaxing music either on its own or while practicing these exercises can be calming.

Exercise

If relaxation is one side of a coin, the flip side of that coin is exercise. Both produce calm and relaxation. Exercise, such as walking, swimming, or lifting weights, helps condition the body as well as build stamina and endurance, which are necessary to counter stress and when using a prosthesis. Exercise also is an excellent for relieving physical and emotional tension that can develop with anxiety or anger.

Balanced Diet

Another strategy is eating a healthy, balanced diet. Too many fats, sweets, or other processed foods may cause individuals to feel run down and fatigued. An unhealthy diet can lead to significant weight gain, which likely affects the ability to wear a prosthesis. As volume increases, sockets do not fit correctly, prompting the need for new sockets to be made, adding to the cost of the prosthesis. In addition, the extra weight on the body has a significant impact on stamina and endurance.

Support from Others

Support from others is an important coping strategy. Having people in amputees' lives is essential for them to rebound from amputations. Those amputees who are able to call on support from spouses, family, and/or friends usually are the most successful at accepting and adapting to amputation. Amputees may dislike becoming dependent on others, which is normal during the early recovery period. Reassurance that this dependency is temporary and that they will learn to do more things on their own helps them feel less guilty and more comfortable reaching out for help.

To receive help from other people, amputees must learn to communicate and share their feelings with others. Amputees can benefit from attending support groups and participating in special programs. The Internet provides access to many Web sites for amputees and people with disabilities, including dating and social networking Web sites. The Amputee Coalition of America offers online support as well as periodic workshops and conferences. Many programs have been developed for amputees who want to engage in physically challenging activities, such as skiing, hiking, and mountain climbing. Some choose to become community activists and advocate for understanding and social/community change. Amputees receive lots of stares but curious children and adults often approach them to ask questions about amputations and their prosthetics. They are in a position to teach others that they are normal and should be treated no different from anyone else.

It also can be annoying when others stare or inquire, which might prompt amputees to become overly aggressive toward others or, alternatively, overly passive or submissive. Encouraging amputees to express their feelings and needs to others as well as teaching them effective communication techniques, such as assertiveness training, can go a long way in helping them get along more effectively with others. Humor helps enable patients to let down their guard. It also tends to disarm others and makes it easier for others to feel comfortable interacting with amputees. Although not a social outlet, journaling is another excellent way to express thoughts and feelings on paper rather than keeping them internalized. Suppressing feelings can cause individuals to ruminate or channel their emotional turmoil into physical tension.

Acceptance

Acceptance of an amputation is crucial to the recovery process. Amputees also need to learn to focus, however, on changing the things they have control over in their lives and letting go of trying to change the things over which they have little or no control. This is the basis of the Serenity Prayer, which many 12-step programs, such as Alcoholics Anonymous, incorporate into their principles and traditions. By focusing on things they can control, amputees can feel empowered. Setting realistic, attainable life and career goals for the future is an example of focusing on the control they have. Returning to work is often a major goal. Amputees can work cooperatively with their employers to modify their workplace to accommodate their disabilities. If they are unable to return to their previous job, they may need to seek vocational rehabilitation services. They may also take the opportunity to change career paths and/or go to school. Often vocational rehab can provide assistance and funding to support retraining.

Many amputees benefit from giving the part of their lives they have little control over to a higher power, such as God. They may believe that their amputation fulfills a mysterious plan that God may have for them. In this way, amputees can feel a sense of meaning in their lives. In general, investment in any activity that provides a sense of purpose or higher meaning—whether in marriage or family, church, or volunteering—helps people feel useful, productive, and worthwhile.

Identifying Negative Self-Talk

Developing awareness of self-talk, the conversations a person has in his or her mind, is a valuable coping skill. Underlying cognitive behavior therapy (CBT) is the belief that negative, unhealthy, maladaptive cognitive patterns (eg, thoughts, beliefs, and attitudes) generate unpleasant emotions, pain, and self-defeating behaviors. The patients whom the authors work with are encouraged to be more aware of their "stinkin' thinkin'" and learn to dispute it by generating more rational, positive thoughts to themselves. Bourne (2011)[6] identified at least 4 distinct voices that characterize negative self-talk: worrier, critic, victim, and perfectionist (**Table 1**).

Table 1
Negative self-talk voices identified by Bourne

Negative Self-Talk	Theme	Common Phrases	Emotions Generated
The worrier	Worries about the worst case scenario	"What if…"	Anxiety
The critic	Self-criticism	"You're such a loser."	Low self-esteem
The victim	Pity party	"Everything's hopeless, so why bother trying to change things?"	Depression
The perfectionist	Need to be perfect and absolutist	"I must always _____ (fill in blank: be perfect, be a pleaser, keep my house clean)."	Disappointment, guilt

Adapted from Bourne E. The anxiety and phobia workbook. 5th edition. Oakland (CA): New Harbinger Publications; 2011.

Patients learn to talk back to such thoughts. For example, a patient who is telling himself, "I'm never going to feel like a whole person again," might say back, "I'm fooling myself if I think I can know what's in store for the future. Let's just focus on the present and let the future unfold whichever way it happens." When patients dispute their negative thinking in this way, they neutralize their thoughts and avoid the unpleasant emotions that normally occur as a result.

EMDR is a technique that incorporates elements of CBT as well as other therapeutic approaches to help patients process and work through the trauma associated with a traumatic injury. It is useful in treating PTSD. EMDR capitalizes on the same rapid eye movement (REM) that occurs when asleep and working through feelings, conflicts, and experiences through dreams. These eye movements help to diminish the power of emotionally charged memories from past traumatic events.[7]

Pacing

Finally, it is important to for patients to pace themselves when engaging in physical activity. Amputees may overdo activities, especially after receiving their prostheses. They may try to take on too much activity at one time and forget to take breaks between activities. The consequence is soreness and swelling in the residual limb. This essentially forces patients to stop wearing the prosthesis for a short period of time to allow the tissue to heal, which can set back their progress. Patients need to learn to live their lives as if they are running a marathon rather than a sprint and to pace themselves throughout the day, giving themselves ample opportunity to conserve their energy by slowing down or even taking rests when appropriate.

Other Helpful Interventions

Patients sometimes need psychiatric and psychopharmacologic interventions as an adjunct to their individual psychotherapy. They often can benefit from an antidepressant or antianxiety medication. Some antidepressants not only improve depression and stabilize mood but also have a positive effect on pain or anxiety. Antianxiety medications (eg, benzodiazepines) should be limited to short-term use because patients often have difficulty getting off of them if used on a long-term basis.

Community reintegration strategies should be incorporated in amputees' care. For example, they should be encouraged to try some volunteer work when they are ready. They can also be steered toward participating in vocational rehabilitation programs for retraining.

DIFFERENCES IN EMOTIONAL HEALING

In discussing positive adaptations to amputation, it would be remiss to not cover individual diversities that may have an impact on outcome: gender, cultural/religious, educational, social support, prior lifestyle, level of functioning, and prior experiences with catastrophes. These are just a few considerations that may need to be explored when assessing and treating patients.

Gender

It is important to assess the female/male role in amputees' lives. Have they been raised predominately with men as the breadwinners and with women more focused on home/family? Loss of limb and possible loss of employment may be devastating to individuals who believe that if they are no longer able to financially support the family, they no longer have any self-worth. Additionally, a former protector may think, "I could not even care for myself, how I can care for my family?" Women raised in families with matriarchs may wonder, "How am I to be respected and keep the family together, if I am not together?"

Gender also plays a role in an individual's body image. The authors' observations are that women are more apt to try and cover-up a prosthesis or look at cosmesis options than are men.

Cultural/Religious Considerations

Cultural/religious considerations are integral to assessing individual personality. In Hispanic cultures, the elder women of the family are frequently consulted on family matters. The men take on the role of breadwinners and the machismo persona. In the treatment of Orthodox Jews, Mennonites, and Mormons, a woman's role is defined as supportive.

Medical care may consist of alternative medical practices. Such cases exist in Native American culture (medicine bags, burning of herbs, and so forth); parts of North America, the Caribbean, and South America and Central American countries (voodoo, use of a *curandero*, and so forth); Africa (local herbalist and doctors); and Asian cultures (acupuncture and so forth). Providing medical care may prove challenging: Middle Eastern and Asian women and members of certain religious groups (Orthodox Jews, Mormons, and so forth) prohibit members of the opposite sex from touching them.

In some cultures and religions, direct eye contact is considered inappropriate, whereas in others direct eye contact is considered a sign of respect and equality. The manner in which men from Middle Eastern or Eastern countries (India and Pakistan) with upper extremity amputations are able to perform basic self-care may be compromised. In several Middle Eastern countries, the right hand is used for eating and the left hand for toileting. Such cultural and religious considerations may have a negative impact on how amputees view themselves.

Age

Individuals with congenital disorders (eg, born without one or more limbs) tend to adapt better emotionally than do those who lose limbs at older ages. As young children learn to crawl, stand, and use their arms for various activities, they learn to adapt to the loss of limb(s) and find other methods to perform tasks. Their self-images incorporate the limb loss. Peers may question why they do not have a particular body part, but as they start to talk, they accept them as they are. In general, children are more resilient to limb loss.

In the teens and early adulthood, amputation becomes more traumatic. Developmentally, teens are developing their personalities and sense of self, and body image is important. Their peers are individuals who think like them and have similar interests, but "are not like them." Amputation at this age is difficult. They may have to redefine themselves at a time when they thought they "knew" who they were. Teens and young adults may be self-deprecating; they may see themselves as ugly or as someone nobody could love. They may wonder who could love someone without a limb(s). Finding a capable therapist to help in address adjustment to disability issues is imperative.

Older patients may find that they need amputation secondary to other medical conditions. They may not seek counseling, because they consider amputation just one more medical problem. Older amputees may be less willing to seek counseling, because they think that this is just something that they need to handle.

Education

It is important to assess an individual's educational level. Information regarding amputation should be presented in terms and language patients can comprehend. Accurate information regarding amputation and the rehabilitation process is imperative to enable an individual to make informed decisions regarding care; however, too much information may increase an individual's stress level and be overwhelming.

Family and Support System Availability

Although a strong family and friend support system is helpful for adapting to amputation, sometimes it can be counterproductive for amputees. An amputee's support system may try to help with various tasks that amputees must learn to do on their own. It is important to counsel amputees as well as the members of their support system on the importance of letting individuals fail in the process of learning to complete tasks. In addition, because the family is going through similar reactions of loss and grief, it is important not to forget the needs of the family. A family may need counseling as much as an amputee.

Prior Lifestyle and Level of Functioning

Knowing how an individual handles stress and uses various coping strategies is important during recovery. Someone who has limited coping strategies before amputation may need to develop new or additional coping strategies. A perfect example is patients who used to run or work out to alleviate stress, who need to develop alternative means to release stress. These patients may have a strong personality that drove them to be competitive in sports; that personality trait may serve them well during the rehabilitation process but also has the potential for doing harm if the patients do not adhere to their prosthetic wearing schedule, believing that they can wear the prosthetic for longer hours than recommended by their physician. This may result in skin breakdown/blisters from overuse.

Prior Life Catastrophes

Some individuals become amputees due to other medical conditions (cancer, diabetes, and so forth), natural catastrophes (earthquakes, tornados, and so forth), or war. Frequently, they feel lucky to be alive. Those who have successfully survived catastrophic events and learned to cope with these catastrophic situations usually have the coping skills necessary to adjust to amputation, although in some cases, individuals with a prior history of life catastrophes may feel victimized. It is important to obtain a psychosocial history to assess and evaluate each individual's specific needs as they pertain to amputation and rehabilitation.

HALLMARKS OF UNSUCCESSFUL EMOTIONAL OUTCOMES OR MALADAPTATION

Some of the factors that indicate an individual is not coping and adapting well after an amputation are discussed. Hopefully, being aware of these variables will enable medical personnel to take action before a patient stops progressing or even relapses.

Pain, Pain, and More Pain

One of the major signs of maladaptation is a high level of pain. Most postamputation pain, including phantom pain, is well controlled through a variety of treatment options, including medications. When an amputee experiences a lot of pain despite receiving appropriate treatment, the focus often becomes the pain itself. Everything else takes a back to seat to trying to control the patient's pain. This can be a perplexing and frustrating experience for both amputees and health care providers. Patients often become overly preoccupied or ruminate about their pain levels, which then become

even further amplified. They may regret choosing the amputation, making it more difficult to accept and adapt to being an amputee.

Anger Outbursts

Patients who struggle with amputation may harbor unresolved anger that they
displace onto their spouses, family, and friends. This can put a terrible strain on relationships, many of which are already stressed from dealing with the amputation
and its consequences. Anger also may be directed toward medical caregivers.
This occurs when patients perceive the cause of their amputations to be negligence,
error, or some other fault caused by their health care professionals. It is often difficult for them to let go of their resentment and blame and they may wonder, "How
could you have let this happen to me?" Patients may question why the doctors
are not able to fix their problems, especially after undergoing amputations, and
may start to doubt their doctors' competence and regret following their advice to
amputate.

Alcohol and Drugs

Using alcohol or illicit drugs to block pain and buffer emotions is a common hallmark of
unsuccessful adaptation to amputation. Self-medication often leads to dependency,
addiction, or abuse. Patients may self-medicate to deaden the pain and loss as well
as mask their feelings of depression, anger, or anxiety. Some use alcohol or drugs
to control these emotions rather than more appropriate medications, such as antidepressants. They likely come from families where self-medicating was the norm or substance abuse was common. They do not realize that although these substances may
work in the short term, they are likely to lead to increased pain, anxiety, or depression
over time. Alcohol, a known depressant, often cancels the benefits of antidepressants
if taken at the same time.

Similarly, some patients abuse prescription medications, especially opiates. Those
who have low pain thresholds may begin to increase their doses beyond amount prescribed because of drug tolerance or wanting complete pain elimination. This may
lead to addiction, using the medication differently from prescribed (eg, smoking or
snorting) or engaging in drug-seeking behaviors, such as doctor shopping. It is common for patients to become dependent on medications and experience physical with-
drawal when they run out or abruptly discontinue taking them.

Negative Outlook on Life

A pessimistic perspective of the future indicates possible problems coping with amputation. This negative orientation about life is frequently a product of feeling bitter,
resentful, or depressed as a result of sustaining an amputation. Those who believe
that life should be more fair or feel entitled to freedom from adversity and suffering
may be disappointed and despairing when things do not work out as hoped. Additionally, those prone to worry or anxiety often anticipate the worst-case scenario
happening in their future—this is known as catastrophizing. A self-fulfilling prophecy
may occur when, believing that their negative expectations will come true, people
somehow create the very circumstances that fulfill their predictions. Thus, if an
amputee believes that he or she will not be able to overcome the amputation, this likely
will prove true.

Lack of Acceptance

It is important to know that some amputees never completely accept their limb loss; it
is too much to believe they can have a fulfilling, enriched lives as amputees. They

continue to yearn and become fixated and preoccupied by their loss. They remain angry and depressed by the unfairness or injustice that has occurred to them and the prospect of being forced to alter their lives so dramatically.

Those with unresolved experiences and trauma in earlier years—such as physical, verbal, emotional, or sexual abuse; loss of a loved one; being bullied or rejected; and alcohol or substance abuse—may find it more difficult to be flexible and adaptable when they undergo an amputation. These experiences may remain dormant for years until such time that trauma associated with an amputation may retrigger these issues and emotions. It is important to understand that these amputees are responding to their amputation not only in the present but also on a deeper level through their experiences from their past. For example, an amputation may be perceived as just another bad thing in a sequence of bad events that have occurred to an individual, reconfirming that "life sucks."

Poor Sleep Pattern

Lack of sleep has a negative impact on progress. Insomnia can result from problems falling or staying asleep due to the effects of pain, discomfort, medications, or sleep apnea. Patients often encounter problems with sleep patterns, sometimes to the point of flipping their awake-sleep schedule. In bed at night, people project their worries and anxieties, and in the quiet and dark, devoid of common daytime distractions, they become captive to their thoughts. Certain medications promote non-REM sleep, which inhibit the restorative REM sleep that is so important to well-being. In a conversation with one of the authors, a physician remarked, "The Geneva Convention outlawed sleep deprivation because it was a form of cruel and inhuman punishment, yet millions of Americans experience sleep deprivation every night." (Paul Leo, MD, personal communication, 2012).

Changes in Appetite and Weight Gain

One factor that causes amputees to stop using their prostheses, and perhaps become less functional or mobile, is body weight variability. Fluctuations in volume can lead to prosthetic sockets not fitting correctly or comfortably. Body weight fluctuations can occur when appetite increases or decreases from pain, anxiety, or depression as well as lack of exercise. Various medications cause a range of negative effects, such as water retention. Narcotics are known to cause constipation and stomach distress, which can affect appetite. Marinol, a derivative of marijuana in pill form, and medicinal marijuana, used often to increase appetite and control pain, also are associated with increased weight.

Not Being Able to Return to Work

The inability to go back to work is another sign of major loss in life. For many men, their work is tied to their sense of identity and self-worth. Not being able to return to their job is not only a career loss but also represents the loss of who they were and how useful they feel. They may think, "I can't do anything anymore," and feel like they no longer have a purpose in life.

On the other hand, fear and anxiety may prevent those who suffered traumatic amputations to avoid returning to work because the workplace is perceived as dangerous and the risk of being injured again seems high. Contemplating returning to work may retrigger PTSD and wanting to avoid bosses and coworkers as well as the machinery associated with their injury. Consequently, they may delay their return as long as possible to avoid feeling overwhelmed and helpless at their worksite.

Lack of Integration into the Community

Amputees may withdraw socially and isolate themselves. They may feel alienated and isolated because they are depressed, are burdened with low self-esteem, or fear how the public will receive them. Every time someone looks at them or stares, they may interpret these actions in a self-referential way and may misperceive people's curiosity as negative judgment and criticism. As a result, they avoid going out in public, preferring to stay home, where they deal with less scrutiny. Unfortunately, avoidance begets avoidance; their world becomes smaller, sometimes to the point where they stop venturing out of their house, bedroom, or even their bed.

HALLMARKS OF SUCCESSFUL EMOTIONAL OUTCOMES AND/OR POSITIVE ADAPTATION TO AMPUTATION

People frequently ask what characterizes successful emotional adaptation to amputation. There are objective and subjective measures for assessing positive adaptation.

Objective Measurements

Prior to amputation surgery or immediately afterward (in cases of traumatic amputation), therapists may ask patients to complete various self-rating questionnaires, to assess signs/symptoms of emotional distress (eg, Beck Depression Inventory). These assessment tools may be administered at regular intervals before and immediately after amputation and throughout the rehabilitation process. Results can be useful tools for assessing the emotional well-being of amputees and determining the best path of treatment.

Subjective Measurements

Communication
Positive emotional outcomes frequently are evident in how amputees interact and communicate with others:

- Is conversation stilted and awkward, or is there a normal flow of communication?
- Are amputees able to assert themselves when necessary (by asking others to provide assistance only when/if asked to do so)?
- Can amputees openly express their feelings?
- Do others in their social circle have to pause and think what they are going to say or avoid certain topics, for fear of making an amputee uncomfortable?
- Can amputees smile and joke about humorous situations pertaining to the amputation (eg, an upper extremity amputee offering to lend a friend hand with a task).
- Can individuals incorporate amputation as part of who they are as persons, or does amputation still define their whole being?

These are all subjective responses in communication that are used as assessment tools to evaluate emotional adaptation.

Return to activities
Quality of life is defined differently for every individual. Those with positive outcomes after amputation are able to have a sense of purpose in their lives. To some, this may mean a return to work, usual family activities, and prior social and community activities, including recreation.

The Road to Successful Adaptation

Positive adaptation may find an amputee advocating for modifications in the work-place, to accommodate for amputation. Some are not be able to return to their pream-putation job and may need to explore a new niche to go with their skill set. Others who find no employment available in their previous workplace may seek out alternate employment or training opportunities through vocational rehabilitation agencies, trade schools, and colleges. People injured on the job may experience PTSD or anxiety around returning to work. Emotional issues must be addressed to successfully transi-tion back to the job. They may have to deal with uneasy coworkers who do not know what to say or how to act.

After amputation, many refrain from family and community activities, either due to their real or perceived inability to physically participate or to changes in their self-images. Amputees may need to find different or modified means to participate in pleasurable activities with people they enjoy. Amputees may need to modify certain activities with equipment, for instance their schedules, because it may take more time to physically complete an activity, or adjust their expectations. Someone who no longer can compete athletically may enjoy participating at a noncompetitive level or coaching others. Families should explore new activities that allow an amputee to participate. Many amputees want to help others who are going through, or have recently undergone, these surgeries. This giving back may take the form of peer counseling, becoming an advocate for other amputees, or participating in support groups.

Satisfactory sexual interaction is an area seldom explored but important to positive adaptation. Is an individual able to become aroused? For men, the issue is the ability to maintain a physical erection. Both men and woman face issues concerning climax/ejaculation: Are they hypersensitive or do they experience pain? Professionals need to assess whether sexual dysfunction is due to physical issues associated with ampu-tation or to emotional issues around self-image. Amputees and their partners may need to broaden their repertoire of stimulation techniques and positions.

Successful emotional outcomes after amputation do not require that amputees no longer think about the circumstances around their amputations or be totally pain-free. The backbone of amputees' positive emotional change is to acknowledge their altered circumstances but not dwell and remain singularly focused on them, to develop coping strategies and the capacity to incorporate their amputee circumstances into their self-concept, or to redefine themselves in ways that acknowledge and accept amputation as part of who they are. In this way, over time, they focus less and less on the ways that amputation dictates how they must live their lives and develop coping strategies that free them to focus on the future and its possibilities.

REFERENCES

1. Kübler-Ross E. On death and dying. New York: Macmillan; 1969.
2. Freud S. Mourning and Melancholia. The standard edition of the complete works of Sigmund Freud. Trans: James Strachy, Vol 14. London: Hogarth Press:Institute of Psychoanalysis; 1953-1974. p. 243–58.
3. American Psychiatric Association (APA). Diagnostic and statistical manual of mental disorders. 5th edition. Washington, DC: American Psychiatric Association; 2013.
4. Zhang B, Maciejewski PK, Prigerson HG, et al. An empirical examination of the stage theory of grief. JAMA 2007;297:716–23.

5. Prigerson HG, Maciejewski PR. Grief and acceptance as opposite sides of the same coin: setting a research agenda to study peaceful acceptance of loss. British Journal of Psychiatry 2008;193:435–7.
6. Bourne E. The anxiety and phobia workbook. 5th edition. Oakland (CA): New Harbinger Publications; 2011.
7. Shapiro F, Forrest MS. EMDR: the breakthrough therapy for overcoming anxiety, stress, and trauma. New York: Basic Books; 1997.

FURTHER READINGS

Baylor College of Medicine. (n.d.). Multicultural patient care: special populations. Available at: http://www.bcm.edu/mpc/special-af.html. Accessed September, 2013.

Behel JM, Rybarczyk B, Elliott TR, et al. The role of perceived vulnerability in adjustment to lower-extremity amputation: a preliminary investigation. Rehabil Psychol 2002;47:92–105.

Bodenheimer C, Kerrigan AJ, Garber SL, et al. Sexuality in persons with lower extremity amputations. Disabil Rehabil 2000;22:409–15.

Bradway JK, Malone JM, Racy J, et al. Psychological adaptation to amputation: an overview. Orthot Prosthet 1984;38(3):46–50.

Breakey JW. Body image: the lower limb amputee. J Prosthet Orthot 1997;9:58–66.

Callaghan B, Condie E, Johnston M. Using the common sense self-regulation model to determine psychological predictors of prosthesis use and activity limitations in lower limb amputees. Prosthet Orthot Int 2008;32:324–36.

Cheung E, Alvaro R, Colotla VA. Psychological distress in workers with traumatic upper- or lower-limb amputations following industrial injuries. Rehabil Psychol 2003; 48:109–12.

Darnall BD, Ephraim P, Wegener ST, et al. Depressive symptoms and mental health service utilization among persons with limb loss. Arch Phys Med Rehabil 2005; 86:650–8.

Desmond DM, MacLachlan M. Coping strategies as predictors of psychosocial adaptation in a sample of elderly veterans with acquired lower limb amputations. Soc Sci Med 2006;62:208–16.

Dise-Lewis JE. Psychological adaption to limb loss. In: Atkins DJ, Meier RH, editors. Comprehensive management of the upper limb amputee. New York: Springer-Verlag; 1989. p. 165–72.

Durance JP, O'Shea BJ. Upper limb amputees: a clinical profile. Disabil Rehabil 1988; 10:68–72.

English AWG. Psychology of limb loss. BMJ 1989;299:1287.

Fran RG, Kashani JH, Kashani SR, et al. Psychological response to amputation as a function of age and time since amputation. Br J Psychiatry 1984;144:493–7.

Friedmann LW. The psychological rehabilitation of the amputee. Springfield (IL): Charles C Thomas Publishers; 1978.

Frierson RL, Lippman SB. Psychiatric consultation for acute amputees. Psychosomatics 1987;28(4):183–9.

Galanti GA. Caring for patients from different cultures. 4th edition. Philadelphia: University of Pennsylvania Press; 2005.

Gallagher P, MacClachlan M. Positive meaning in amputation and thoughts about the amputated limb. Prosthet Orthot Int 2000;24:196–204.

Gerhards F, Floren I, Knapp T. The impact of medial re-educational and psychological variable on rehabilitation outcome in amputees. Int J Rehabil Res 1984;7(3):283–92.

Green MM, McFarlance AC, Hunter CE, et al. Undiagnosed post-traumatic stress disorder following motor vehicle accidents. Med J Aust 1993;159(8):529–34.

Grunert BK, Divine CA, Maloub HS, et al. Psychological adjustment following work-related hand injury: 18-month follow-up. Ann Plast Surg 1992;29(6):537–42.

Ham R, Regan JM, Roberts VC. Evaluation of introducing the team approach to the care of the amputee: the Dulwich Study. Prosthet Orthot Int 1987;11:25–30.

Hamill R, Carson S, Dorahy M. Experiences of psychosocial adjustment within 18 months of amputation: an interpretative phenomenological analysis. Disabil Rehabil 2010;32:729–40.

Hamilton A. Rehabilitation of the leg amputee in the community. Practitioner 1981;225:1487.

Hill A, Niven CA, Knussen C, et al. Rehabilitation outcome in long-term amputees. Br J Ther Rehabil 1995;2:593–8.

Horgan O, Maclachlan M. Psychosocial adjustment to lower limb amputation: a review. Disabil Rehabil 2004;26:837–50.

Juckett G. Cross cultural medicine. Am Fam Physician 2005;72(11):2267–74.

Kashani JH, Frank RG, Kashani SR, et al. Depression among amputees. J Clin Psychiatry 1983;44:256–8.

Kohl SJ. Psychosocial stressors in coping with disability. In: Krieger DW, editor. Rehabilitation psychology: a comprehensive textbook. Rockville (MD): Aspen Systems Corporation; 1984. p. 113–48.

Marks L. Lower limb amputees: advantages of the team approach. Practitioner 1987;231:1321–4.

Martz E, Cook DW. Physical impairments as risk factors for the development of post-traumatic stress disorder. Rehabil Couns Bull 2001;44:217–21.

Meichenbaum D. A clinical handbook/practical therapist manual for assessing and treating adults with posttraumatic stress disorder (PTSD). Waterloo (Ontario): Institute Press; 1994.

Nicholas JJ, Robinson LR, Schulz R, et al. Problems experienced and perceived by prosthetic patients. J Prosthet Orthot 1993;5:16–9.

Nissen SJ, Newman WP. Factors influencing reintegration to normal living after amputation. Arch Phys Med Rehabil 1992;73:548–61.

Paniagua FA. Assessing and treating culturally diverse clients: a practical guide. 3rd edition. Thousand Oaks (CA): Sage Publications Inc; 2005.

Pfefferbaum B, Pasnau RO. Post-amputation grief. Nurs Clin North Am 1976;11(687):690.

Phelps LF, Williams RM, Raichle A, et al. The importance of cognitive processing to adjustment in the 1st year following amputation. Rehabil Psychol 2008;53(1):28–38.

Price EM, Fisher KD. How does counseling help people with amputation? J Prosthet Orthot 2002;14:102–8.

Price EM, Fisher KD. Additional studies of the emotional needs of amputees. J Prosthet Orthot 2005;17:52–6.

Rybarczyk BD, Nyenhuis DL, Nicholas JJ, et al. Social discomfort and depression in a sample of adults with leg amputations. Arch Phys Med Rehabil 1992;73:1169–73.

Rybarczyk BD, Nyenhuis DL, Nicholas JJ, et al. Body image, perceived social stigma, and the prediction of psychosocial adjustment to leg amputation. Rehabil Psychol 1995;40:95–110.

Rybarczyk B, Edwards R, Behel J. Diversity in adjustment to a leg amputation: case illustrations of common themes. Disabil Rehabil 2004;26:944–53.

Saradjian A, Thompson AR, Datta D. The experience of men using an upper limb prosthesis following amputation: positive coping and minimizing feeling different. Disabil Rehabil 2008;30:871–83.

Shukla GD, Sahu SC, Tripathi RP, et al. A psychiatric study of amputees. Br J Psychiatry 1982;28:183–9.

Singh R, Hunter J, Philip A. The rapid resolution of depression and anxiety symptoms after lower limb amputation. Clin Rehabil 2007;21(8):754–9.

Smurr LM, Gulick K, Yancosek K, et al. Managing the upper extremity amputee: a protocol for success. J Hand Ther 2008;21:160–75.

Thompson DM, Haran D. Living with an amputation: what it means for patients and their helpers. Int J Rehabil Res 1984;7:283–93.

Unwin J, Kacperek L, Clark C. A prospective study of positive adjustment to lower limb amputation. Clin Rehabil 2009;23:1044–50.

Van Dorsten B. Integrating psychological and medical care: practice recommendations for amputation. In: Meier RH, Atkins DJ, editors. Functional restoration of adults and children with upper extremity amputation. New York NYC(NY): Demos Medical Publishing; 2004. p. 73–88.

Wald J, Alvaro R. Psychological factors in work related amputation: considerations for rehabilitation counselors. J Rehabil 2004;70:96–102.

Whyte A, Carroll LJ. The relationship between catastrophizing and disability in amputees experiencing phantom pain. Disabil Rehabil 2004;26:649–54.

Willamson GM, Schulz R, Bridges MS, et al. Social and psychological factors in adjustment to limb amputation. J Soc Behav Pers 1994;9:249–68.

Winchell E. Coping with limb loss: a practical guide to living with amputation for you and your family. Garden City Park (NY): Avery Publishing Group; 1995.

Wortman C, Silver R. The myths of coping with loss. J Consult Clin Psychol 1989;57:349–57.

Amputee Rehabilitation and Preprosthetic Care

Julie Klarich, OTR, CHT*, Inger Brueckner, PT

KEYWORDS

- Occupational therapy intervention • Upper and lower extremity amputee
- Prosthesis • Preprosthetic training • Physical therapy intervention
- Treatment of phantom limb pain • Physical therapy • Exercise

KEY POINTS

- The occupational therapist can contribute important information to the team in deciding the proper prescription for the prosthesis.
- The functional goals of the patient in using the prosthesis should be acknowledged in planning the prosthetic components.
- Vocational and avocational needs should also be taken into consideration.
- The amputation surgery is just the start of a long, arduous process to get the patient back to as many of their previous activities as possible.
- The most vital participation in the whole process is the amputee's participation.
- There are several exercise programs that can be integrated in between amputation surgery and prosthetic delivery that can improve outcomes for patients.

OCCUPATIONAL THERAPY INTERVENTION FOR PREPROSTHETIC TRAINING IN THE LOWER EXTREMITY AMPUTEE
General Evaluation

The occupational therapy evaluation for a lower extremity amputee should include assessment of upper extremity (UE) range of motion (ROM) and strength, including grip and pinch strength. Lower limb amputees will need to use crutches or propel a wheelchair before prosthetic fit. Upper extremity weakness or injury can impact the ability to ambulate with these assistive devices. Sensory deficits in the upper extremities can be due to injury or preexisting cumulative trauma, from after chemotherapy, or from diabetic neuropathy. Endurance compared with previous level of function should be noted because it requires more energy to walk with a prosthesis. Core strength and general conditioning are also very important in achieving the optimal level of function and are especially important if the amputee has been hospitalized for a long period of time.

Presbyterian/St. Luke's Medical Center, Outpatient Rehabilitation Center, 1601 East, 19th Avenue Suite 6100, Denver, CO 80218, USA
* Corresponding author.
E-mail address: Julie.klarich@healthonecares.com

Phys Med Rehabil Clin N Am 25 (2014) 75–91
http://dx.doi.org/10.1016/j.pmr.2013.09.005
1047-9651/14/$ – see front matter © 2014 Elsevier Inc. All rights reserved.

Evaluation of Activities of Daily Living

A comprehensive activity of daily-living evaluation should be completed including evaluation of the home. It is important to note the number of steps for entry and exit of the home. A ramp may be indicated if the patient will return home in a wheelchair. If it is a 2-level home, then arrangements can be made for living on the main level or a stair glide or elevator can be installed. These arrangements are usually only indicated for bilateral lower extremity amputees or medically compromised individuals. The bathroom is a common place for falls. It is usually recommended for there to be a shower chair or transfer bath bench as well as grab rails for bathing. Some amputees will need a raised or higher toilet seat and/or bars next to the toilet for push off during standing. The patient should be educated to remove all throw rugs as they are easy to trip on in the home. A nonskid mat should be used in the bottom of the bath or shower. A hand-held shower is helpful in control of the water from a seated position. If the bathroom doorway is too narrow for a wheelchair to pass through, then the patient may enter with crutches or sideways with a walker. A transfer wheelchair is often narrow enough to navigate through the doorway because it does not have the outside wheels.

Evaluation for Driving

If the patient has had amputation of both lower limbs or the right leg, then adaptation may need to be completed for driving. Many right transtibial amputees (TTA) are still able to drive with their prosthesis; however, a left foot accelerator or hand controls can also be used for safety. An evaluation with a certified adapted driving instructor is recommended.

Occupational Therapy Treatment of Lower Extremity Amputees

Activities of daily living

All adaptive equipment for home safety should be ordered or purchased by the family and properly installed. At times a home evaluation is indicated to identify the safety needs of the client properly. Instruction should be given in homemaking activities from the wheelchair level or crutches as indicated.

Therapeutic exercise

Maximizing UE strength, core strength, and endurance will greatly help lower extremity amputees with function during activities of daily living (ADL) and in transitioning to prosthetic use.

PREPROSTHETIC CARE FOR THE UE AMPUTEE
Preoperative Care

When it is possible to see a patient before amputation, it is helpful to evaluate the patient for the status of the limb and the possible goals in having the limb amputated. Occupational therapy can assist in helping to determine the optimal level of amputation for function as well as helping to determine the functional outcome goals for having the amputation performed.

Evaluation

The comprehensive evaluation should include the following:

- Assessment of ROM of all joints
- Strength of the entire upper quadrant
- Pain level and cause of pain
- Sensation of the limb

- Current ADL function of the patient
- Psychological and social support
- Vocation and avocation needs.

Treatment

- ADL training should include instruction in one-handed techniques and adaptive equipment that may be helpful at the time and/or after amputation. Dominance retraining can begin at this stage and assist in the transition for change of dominance if it is the dominant hand that will be amputated. ROM of both upper extremities should be maximized before surgery. There should be careful focus on scapulothoracic motion as well. All individuals will also benefit from maximizing UE strength, core strength, and endurance.

Team Collaboration

- The occupational therapy evaluation can give useful information to the patient and the team in deciding the level of amputation as well as whether amputation will improve function for an individual. For example, if muscle testing reveals weak bicep function, the patient may not benefit from a transradial amputation because the weight of the prosthesis would make it difficult or impossible to bend the elbow. A patient may be considering amputation due to limited function of an extremity, but may have unrealistic expectations of the capabilities of prosthetics. It then becomes the responsibility of the team to educate the patient in the functional abilities of prosthetics.

Postoperative care

- For many individuals, the period of time immediately after an amputation can be a difficult one. Patients may have questions about what they will be able to do. Will they be able to drive, return to work, be accepted by their family and friends? Information and reassurance about return to activity with or without a prosthesis is critical at this time for the amputee and their family. Referral to a support group and/or individual counseling may be appropriate. Early treatment after surgery should include incision/wound care, active ROM of the residual limb and sound limb, ADL training in one-handed techniques and equipment, if it was not already done preoperatively, edema control, and pain management.

Preprosthetic training for the UE amputee

During this phase of treatment, it is important to educate the patient on the process of preparing the residual limb for the prosthesis. A home program should be established for ROM, scar mobilization, desensitization, and volume reduction.

Shaping and Shrinking

- Once the sutures have been removed, shaping and shrinking the limb can be initiated and can be accomplished with figure-of-8 wrapping (**Fig. 1**), use of a shrinker, or a compressive stockinette. If the residual limb has a bulbous end or invagination in the skin, then the figure-of-8 wrap may be the best choice, because you can control the direction of pull and the amount of tension on each area of the limb. The amputee can be taught to wrap the limb themselves by holding the end of the ace wrap down with the residual limb until it is secure or using tape to hold it. Wrapping should be performed distal to proximal with decreasing amount of tension as the wrap is brought proximal to guide the edema out of the distal limb. To main constant compression, it is recommended

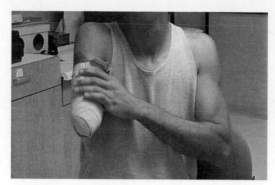

Fig. 1. Figure-of-8 wrapping.

that the figure-of-8 wrap be rewrapped every 4 hours. Compression should be worn at all times except for showering. Multiple wraps should be issued to allow for washing daily.

Posture Training

- Most new amputees will hold the shoulder on the affected side higher or lower than the sound side shoulder. Observation in the mirror and frequent cues to correct posture will often help the amputee to begin self-correction and improve balance.[1]

Desensitization

- Hypersensitivity of the residual limb is common after amputation. The patient should be encouraged to touch the limb and rub the limb with various textures of material to help desensitize it. Light massage and tapping are also helpful. Running the limb through a tub of rice, beans, or macaroni is a useful home program activity.[2]

Scar Management

- Once the incision and all wounds are healed, it is important to ensure that all tissue on the residual limb is mobile. If scar is adherent, then this could be an area of friction in the socket and cause a blister or skin breakdown to occur. Scar massage and silicone or fabricated scar pads can be useful in mobilizing scar. The patient should be educated in scar massage as part of the home program.[1]

ROM

- At this time it is critical to maximize ROM of both upper extremities. Special attention should be paid to internal and external rotation for the transhumeral amputee and forearm supination and pronation for the transradial amputee. These motions will be essential for positioning the prosthesis for function. A transhumeral residual limb that is more than two-thirds the length below the elbow may be able to supinate and pronate to position the prosthesis. Transhumeral amputees can use internal and external rotation to position the terminal device toward midline or away from the body for daily activity. Scapular mobility is also very important for use with cable-operated prostheses. Limited shoulder mobility makes donning and doffing of a prosthesis difficult if there is a harness. Adaptations may be made to the harness for independent donning and doffing.

Pain Management

- During the initial occupational therapy evaluation, it should be established whether pain is in the residual limb or phantom limb. The patient should understand the distinction between phantom pain and phantom sensation. Phantom sensation can be present and not painful. Initially decreasing edema and sensitivity can be helpful in reducing pain. Electrical stimulation such as transcutaneous electrical nerve stimulation, interferential, and high-volt pulsed galvanic stimulation can all be used for pain.[3] If use of the electric stimulation is helpful in the clinic, then a home unit can be obtained to manage pain at home and reduce the use of pain medication. Mirror therapy is another useful tool in managing pain.[4,5] Mirror therapy is a technique in which the amputee is positioned so that they are holding their sound hand in front of a mirror and the amputated limb is hidden behind the mirror. The patient then performs a series of movements in the mirror while watching what appears to be both hands moving through the range of movement. It is important that the patient is educated in the purpose of this treatment and the need for consistency in the home program. The patient is asked to complete this exercise 5 times per day for 15 minutes. Exercises should continue for 1 month. If their pain is increased by the mirror therapy, then they should decrease the intensity of the motion and possibly the frequency. The treatment is discontinued if pain continues to be elevated (**Fig. 2**).

Strengthening of UEs

- Strengthening of the residual limb should not begin until the surgeon thinks that there is sufficient healing to provide resistance safely without compromising the surgical tissues. Progress from gentle isometrics to resistive exercise such as cuff weights on the residual limb and use of theraband to gain strength usually begins after clearance by the physician.

Conditioning and Endurance Training

- Conditioning and endurance training is covered later in the physical therapy section, but general conditioning of core strength, balance, and endurance are essential to the optimal outcome after this type of devastating injury and is especially true for bilateral UE amputees. They will need to have maximal mobility of the cervical and thoracic spine, as well as mobility of the hips to complete ADL.

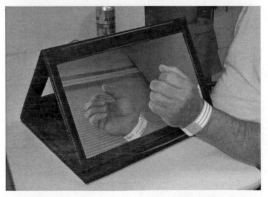

Fig. 2. During the initial occupational therapy evaluation, it should be established whether pain is in the residual limb or phantom limb.

ADL

- Dominance retraining should begin early if the amputated limb was the dominant hand before injury. This training can include writing practice, instruction in position of the paper, and fine-motor coordination activities. Instruction in one-handed techniques and adaptive equipment for independence in ADL is important at this stage. Every amputee should be independent in daily activity without the prosthesis because the amputee may choose not to wear the prosthesis at all times or it may not be available due to breakage or repairs. Education in one-handed shoe tie (**Fig. 3**) and use of the residual limb to stabilize objects is useful. Adaptive equipment can be helpful to some people for ease in completing daily activities. It is important to assess what the patient is having difficulty with and explore options to make the task easier. At times the patient just needs to learn a new way of doing things, but sometimes an adapted aid can make things go faster. Some examples of this equipment are elastic shoelaces, suction nailbrush, electric can opener, rocker knife, and adapted cutting board. Many amputees can drive with little or no adaptation; however, this may need to be assessed by a qualified driving evaluator especially if the amputee has lost both limbs. It is important to identify the goals of the patient for return to work and/or avocational activities. Many sports activities like skiing and swimming can be accomplished without prostheses. Prosthetic adaptations are available for recreational activities and the amputee should be educated in these as appropriate.

Myoelectric Site Testing/Training

- The occupational therapist (OT) can assist in identifying if the residual limb has viable muscle activity for fitting with a myoelectric prosthesis. The sites can be identified manually, with a myotester biofeedback unit. This device detects biofeedback from the muscle activity in the residual limb. It is ideal to have 2

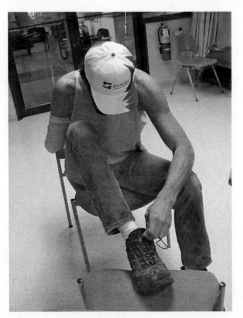

Fig. 3. One-handed shoe tie.

control sites, but a myoelectric prosthesis can be controlled with one site as well. The usual sites for transhumeral level are the bicep for the close signal and the tricep for the open signal. At the transradial level the usual sites are the wrist extensors for the open signal and the wrist flexors for the close signal. At any level the myoelectric site generally needs to be within the socket of the prosthesis. For partial hand prostheses these signals may be in the small muscles of the hand or touch pads may be used with the remnant digits.

- Once the myoelectric signals have been identified, training may need to take place to increase the strength of these muscles or work on patterns of muscle activity that can be used to program the various prehension patterns of the terminal device and/or switch between elbow, wrist, and hand function.

Preprosthetic Training for Bilateral Upper Extremity Amputees

- It is important to provide some sense of independence to the bilateral UE amputee as early as possible after injury. A touch pad call light in the hospital room is important so that the patient can get help when needed. The dominant residual limb can be fitted with a universal cuff. Objects can be inserted into the cuff for use with feeding, brushing teeth, writing, and controlling the television in the room. Foot skills for the bilateral UE amputee can be useful in manipulating their environment. Feet can be useful in opening doors, putting socks on, and a variety of activities. Flexibility in the hips and dexterity in the toes will help determine the usefulness of the feet for assisting in task completion. It is important that patients at this level be educated in using their whole body during ADL. Objects can be picked up with the chin to the chest, the hip can be used against the countertop to hold an object steady, and objects can be held between the residual limb and the side of the body, are all ways that the body can be used for ADL.
- Adaptations for ADL and adaptive equipment for the bilateral arm amputee are vital to gaining independence. Transradial and long transhumeral amputees can often manage quite well by using their residual limbs together to accomplish tasks.

Bathing

- A self-soaping sponge system can be installed in the shower for independent washing. Use of a shower chair or bath bench can help the patient use feet and knees to assist in bathing. A wash mitt can be applied to the residual limb and pushbutton soap dispensers installed as well. Towels can be adapted by folding the end in and sewing pockets for the residual limbs. Body dryers are available that can be installed. Other techniques that are helpful are donning a terrycloth robe after showering or laying towels on the bed and rolling around on the towel for drying. Lever-style knobs on faucets allow for ease in turning on the water and controlling the temperature of the water.

Toileting

- Before prosthetic fit, toileting can be a daunting task. For high-level bilateral arm amputees, a bidet is recommended for ease with toileting at home. All amputees should be taught techniques that can be used when away from home. Placing a pile of toilet paper on the rim of the toilet with the tail of the paper in the water then rubbing the buttocks on the paper can be effective. Flushable wipes can assist in thorough cleaning. The heel of the foot can also be used in this way if the patient has the flexibility to touch the heel of the foot to the buttocks. Clothing management after toileting can be accomplished using the residual limbs inside elastic waist pants to pull the pants up. Patients should be advised to purchase looser fitting clothing, as tight clothing is too difficult to manage.

Dressing

- T-shirts can be pulled over the head by putting the residual limbs into the sleeves and then pulling the shirt over the head and down. A dressing tree can be fashioned using a 2 × 4 board or poly(vinyl chloride) pipe with bicycle hooks at strategic levels for pulling pants up and down as well as helping to don shirts and socks (**Fig. 4**).
- A Dycem mat on the floor can provide enough friction to assist in sliding socks on using toes to hold sock open.
- Slip-on shoes or shoes with Velcro closure are easiest. Elastic laces can be used as well.

Grooming

- An electric razor is safer for shaving for a bilateral arm amputee. For high-level bilateral amputees, a tabletop microphone stand can be used to hold a razor, electric toothbrush, or comb. An electric toothpaste dispenser aids in getting toothpaste onto the brush.
- A small vise on the bathroom countertop can be used to hold deodorant.

Eating

- Initially a plate guard or scoop dish makes getting food onto the fork easier. A swivel spoon or spork can be used to keep the utensil level. The patient should bring their face close to the table to make getting the food to the mouth easier. The fork or spoon can be placed in a universal cuff on the residual limb.

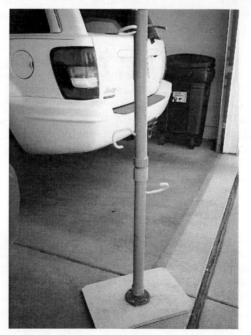

Fig. 4. A dressing tree.

Food Preparation

- Dicing and chopping can be difficult for bilateral amputees. A small chopper or food processor can make this task easier. An electric can opener and jar opener can also be useful. Purchasing prepared food such as grated cheese is recommended. Patients should be educated to store food in easy-to-open containers. The microwave should be located on the countertop for easy access. Instruction can be given on sliding objects along the countertop or using a cart to transport objects if they are heavy or hot.

Home Modifications

- It is important that the bilateral amputee can safely enter and exit the home. Lever-style handles make opening doors easier for interior and exterior doors. A keyless entry eliminates having to use a key. For bilateral amputees voice activation can be used for lights, television, and control of electronics. Voice activation can also be used for computer function and cell phone.

Occupational Therapy's Role in Prosthetic Prescription

The OT can contribute important information to the team in deciding the proper prescription for the prosthesis. The functional goals of the patient in using the prosthesis should be acknowledged in planning the prosthetic components. Vocational and avocational needs should also be taken into consideration. At times the patient may need to have more than one prosthesis to accomplish all of the functional goals. Ultimately it is extremely important for the amputee to be central in the final decision about the prosthetic prescription. Concerns about cosmesis, social acceptance, function, and durability should all be considered.

PHYSICAL THERAPY PREPROSTHETIC REHABILITATION OF LOWER EXTREMITY AND UE AMPUTEES

The amputation surgery is just the start of a long, arduous process to get the patient back to as many of their previous activities as possible. Often patients are seen who have struggled, enduring months to years of attempts at limb salvage, only to feel like they, and the medical team, "failed" when there is an amputation. The program outlined here includes treatment of amputees before prosthetic training that is performed in the authors' hospital. There is a lack of high-quality studies on the specifics of the rehabilitation program in the preprosthetic phase for all of the different types of amputees. Included in this article are some of the clinical choices the authors' team has made based on their experience treating hundreds of amputees. The authors' approach is multidisciplinary and includes face-to-face interaction on a regular basis to meet the needs of the patient. Both physical therapist (PT) and OT see every patient, regardless if they are an upper or lower extremity amputee.

The goal is to make every amputee as functional as possible in or out of their prosthetics. It is hoped that all patients use their prosthetics to the best of their ability. However, it is understood that not everyone will become a prosthetic user. It is important that they have the best available training so they can make an informed decision on what is the right for them. Each individual rehabilitation program is developed so that the patient is as successful as possible.

The amputee population is at great risk. The 5-year mortality after new-onset diabetic ulceration has been reported to be between 43% and 74% for patients with lower extremity amputation. These mortalities can be higher than those for several types of cancer including prostate, breast, and colon, and Hodgkin disease.[6] There is evidence that a rehabilitation program can improve mortality in amputees.[7] The experienced amputee rehabilitation team must be aware of the how much risk this population has. The patient can become very deconditioned, while every attempt to save the limb or the life of the patient is made. Even if the patient is not a prosthetic candidate, they could benefit from amputee rehabilitation.

The rehabilitation process can begin preamputation. If the patient presents preoperatively, the patient's current medical status is reviewed; the home environment is looked at, and mobility needs such as wheelchair, crutches, walker, and bathroom modifications, ROM, strength, and endurance are also reviewed.

Exercises are started preoperatively that will allow a more seamless transition from the hospital and can include isometrics, postural exercises, balance exercises, stretching, core stability, and UE exercise and resistive exercise. ADLs such as transfers, crutch, walker, or wheelchair use are worked on along with mobility exercises. Review of the therapy treatment plan and expected outcomes can alleviate some anxiety in the patient and/or family. Unfortunately, the individual's insurance coverage is very important in developing a comprehensive treatment plan from surgery to mastering a prosthesis. Other factors to consider when making a rehabilitation plan include the patient's transportation needs, the ability to commit to therapy appointments, and additional medical appointments that will be needed after surgery for other medical issues.

Immediately after the amputation, a thorough physical therapy evaluation is essential. The specific physical therapy evaluation for the amputee after surgery is outlined well in Physical Rehabilitation:

History
Systems review
Skin
Residual limb
Emotional status
Vasuclarity
ROM
Muscle strength
Neurologic
Functional status[8,9]

Because the authors use a multidisciplinary team, they try to share information during the team evaluation to avoid duplication.

The inpatient stay can vary significantly based on the patient's health, level of function, available help at home, and insurance coverage. Patients present who have been discharged home after an outpatient transradial amputation, discharged home from the acute care hospital, discharged to a rehabilitation hospital, or discharged to a skilled nursing facility. Multilimb amputees stay in the hospital for months, or patients can be in and out of the hospital for months. The outlined treatment plan below can occur in the hospital, in the home, in the rehabilitation hospital, or in an outpatient setting depending on the needs and medical status of the patient at the time.

Initially postoperatively, the therapist starts the patient with transfer training, limb positioning, and mobility with a focus on household independence. The entire rehabilitation team works to coordinate on the components of ADLs such as bathing, dressing, ambulation, and wheelchair use.

Positioning is addressed with the patient from postoperative day 1. The patient needs to understand the risk of contractures. Most TTA are fitted with a protective cover that also keeps the knee straight. It can be uncomfortable for the patient who has very tight hamstrings. It is difficult and very painful to gain knee extension in a trans-tibial amputation as well as hip extension in the transfemoral amputee (TFA) if they develop a contracture. Often the older, diabetic, and/or vascular patient may have a knee or hip contraction before the amputation. Patient and family education as well as regular follow-up is necessary in preventing contractures. The presence of contractures negatively impacts the ambulatory outcome for the patient.[8]

In the authors' hospital there is a wide variety of dressing types and protocols. The patient can be in a cast, a rigid removable dressing, a wound VAC, and ace bandage or a soft wound dressing. The medical plan of the orthopedic surgeon tends to be different than the vascular surgeon or the plastic surgeon. If there is a physiatrist on the medical team, the therapist relies on him to determine the rehabilitation treatment plan.

Safety should be addressed early after surgery. These patients can very ill and unable to assess the risk and transfer safely. More frequently than imaginable, the patient, gets up, groggy from medication, has enough phantom sensation to think the limb is still present, and falls. A fall on the healing residual limb can be devastating. The patient and family need to understand the real danger of a fall. Gait aides and wheelchair should be periodically assessed to ensure they continue to be the most appropriate device.

Mortalities in diabetic and nondiabetic amputees are high. However, diabetic amputees undergo contralateral amputations and revisions more often than other amputees. Foot ulceration even in the absence of any microvascular complication is associated with higher mortality rates in patients with diabetes.[10] Care of the sound limb is as important as managing the residual limb in the diabetic and vascular patient. Diabetic foot care principles must be followed for all of amputee patients. Routine foot care to protect the sound limb must start as soon as the patient enters rehabilitation. The foot should be examined, washed, and dried daily including in between the toes, and the patient with diabetes should wear proper, well-fitting shoes indoors and outdoors. Autonomic dysfunction will make the plantar aspect of the heel prone to cracks, and the patient should avoid tight socks and put on clean socks every day.[8] Slippers and Croc-type footwear may be wider and easier for the patient to don, but they do not provide the correct support and protection needed. Many amputees use poor footwear and are reluctant to change.

As soon as the surgeon gives clearance, the residual limb is moved and scar healing and mobility are monitored. The patient should begin visual inspection, wound management, and desensitization techniques once they have access to the residual limb. The surgeons or physiatrists determine when to start compression of the residual limb. Ideally, the patient is in compression for 23 of the 24 hours while at home for a minimum of 2 weeks before being casted for a prosthesis (**Fig. 5**).

There are several types of compression: shrinkers, tube-a-grip, and wrapping all with minimal evidence in the literature for comparable effectiveness.[11] The type of compression should be individualized for the patient. For example: the vascular amputee with visual deficits and limited mobility may be unable reach or see the residual limb to wrap safely, but may be able to don a shrinker. The diabetic amputee with significant peripheral neuropathy in their hands may not have the grip strength to pull on a shrinker that has appropriate compression. The therapist needs to monitor the patient's compression use and effectiveness regularly as well as the current limb shape. Effective compression will change the shape of the limb, and as the changes occur, the current method may need to be modified. The skin of the entire residual limb needs to be inspected daily (or more frequently if there are areas of risk) to avoid breakdown with compression or poorly applied compression.

Scar tissue, skin grafts, and radiated skin can all become adherent and at risk for breakdown. Radiated tissue can continue to scar down for 18 months after application

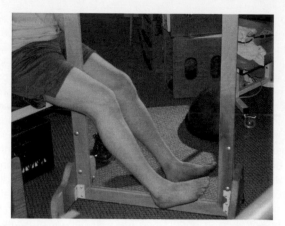

Fig. 5. An inspection mirror.

and should be monitored. Scar tissue is particularly susceptible to sheer forces and may become an area of breakdown or discomfort in compression, or later on in the prosthesis. Communication of the prosthetic plan and medical concerns among the care providers are crucial to avoid setback in the early stage.

The authors begin scar mobilization once the medical team gives the approval. While performing scar mobilization, the scar should be watched for blanching and areas of adhesion. If the patient has increased scar sensitivity to light touch, using a variety of textures can help; there are several examples of desensitization techniques in the therapy literature. The patient may find contraction of the muscles under the scar along with gentle scar mobility can be less painful and more effective than just scar mobility alone.

The authors begin contraction of the residual muscles as soon as the surgeon allows. They take into consideration if the muscle was reattached with a myodesis or a myoplasty. They also use pain as a limit to the force of the contraction early on. TTAs that are able to ambulate in the community will contract the stump musculature in the socket. The timing is not the same for the muscles in a sound limb, but at full volitional recruitment.[12,13] The TFA also contracts the muscles of the residual limb in the socket while ambulating. It is thought that contraction of the musculature in the stump helps with venous return, assists with proprioceptive feedback, and improves stability in the socket during amputation. A very small study showed that an amputee could increase strength and volume in residual muscles with a training program.[14,15]

The authors see Ertl or transtibial osteomyoplastic amputation at their facility. There are specifically designed distal compression exercises that begin at 4 weeks and work up to progressive distal end weight-bearing. If they are done appropriately, the patient often reports the limb feels better after compression/weight-bearing. The Ertl program also advocates early mobility of the sciatic and femoral nerves to avoid nerve adhesions.[14]

A big focus of PT and OT rehabilitation after amputation is cardiovascular exercise. One patient claimed (after a 3-month hospitalization for multiple complications of diabetes) that he was not "weak as a kitten"' but "weak as a gerbil on its death bed.". Aerobic exercise to gain endurance for ADLs is clearly important. The new amputee needs to be very closely monitored during aerobic activity. The authors routinely monitorheart rate, O_2 saturation levels, blood pressure, blood glucose, and perceived exertion rate. The authors also train the patient to monitor their exercise response independently as well. The authors find that sometimes the patient is so deconditioned that getting ready for rehabilitation (getting showered, dressed, and transported) takes all the energy they have. Their initial response to outpatient therapy can be poor if they are not educated and monitored. Often the patient with long-term diabetes does not sense signs of low glucose. Because the patient with diabetes is at such high risk, the authors had the diabetes education department in-service the department on multiple occasions so they can provide safe, appropriate exercise with this group and recognize the risk factors. Critically ill patients also have cardiovascular risk with exercise and need similar monitoring of tolerance of the activity.

The authors try to provide a variety of cardiovascular exercises to avoid overuse and boredom. They have found the NuStep can accommodate patients that have limited mobility. Elastic tubing, the Bosu and exercise ball, arm ergometer, and aquatic therapy can increase heart rate. Endurance, as well as core strength, is needed for all ADLs. The authors use occupational therapy and physical therapy to achieve goals. Physical therapy is more commonly thought to provide cardiovascular exercise and core strength, are a part of both discipline's therapy goals, and can be addressed. Other activities that either therapist can perform include wound care, scar mobility, desensitization, ROM, balance, and weight shift. By having the OT and PT involved, the treatment plan can be more flexible, address more concerns in a given timeframe, and prepare the patient better for prosthetic success. The authors' appointments are typically 1 hour and no single therapy can address all of the needs of our amputees so they have an hour of both.

Traumatic lower extremity amputees also have increased morbidity and mortality from cardiovascular disease. Risk factors include proximal amputation greater than distal, bilateral greater than unilateral, even after body mass index and comorbidities are taken into consideration. There is some concern about hemodynamic consequences of the amputation as well as insulin resistance and psychological stress.[16–18]

Mobility and exercise are difficult and there is often balancing to avoid cumulative trauma of the joints that remain and maximizing efficiency of those limbs.[19] The authors' hospital has a warm water pool and they have found aquatic exercise, once all wounds are healed, is a great option for the patient. The patients have reported having greater ease of all motion, particularly the trunk, in the water instead of the mat. The authors try to have everyone try the water whather they are a TTA, hemipelvectomy, or quadruple amputee. For the patient who has many injuries or illnesses that prevent early fit of prosthetics, they can be upright in the pool, float, and have more control of trunk motion than some traditional mat exercises can afford. There is also very low impact with aquatic exercise.

Hip extension is very important to gain and maintain particularly in TFA. The patient will often bring the residual limb posterior to the trunk using lumbar extension and an anterior pelvic tilt, not true hip extension. Controlling excessive anterior pelvic tilt can be very hard for the patient and the therapist. The authors attempt to have all of their amputees spend time prone: for example, 20 minutes in the morning and 20 minutes in the evening daily. This is not always possible especially in the geriatric amputee. An alternate technique is to hold the sound limb in hip and knee flexion to capture the pelvis and decrease anterior tilt and then bring the residual limb toward the mat table or bed, if at home.

Hip extensor strength is a strong predictor of mobility in a 6-minute walk test for amputees and weakness is a strong contributor to gait abnormalities.[20] The amputee needs hip strength to absorb ground reaction force and to propel the limb.[21] A practical understanding of the forces and muscle action that the amputee uses for gait is an integral part of planning exercise in the preprosthetic phase of rehabilitation.[13,22] For the TFA, hip extension, abduction, and core stability play a vital role in mobility. For the TTA, they co-contract the hamstring and quadriceps as well as initiate walking from the hip musculature. Hip strength is also important in the sound limb.

The lower extremity amputee can be prone to median nerve issues.[23] A small study by Pyo and colleagues reported 80% of the patients had positive electromyogram findings with neuropathy at the wrist and 70% at the elbow of long-term lower extremity amputees. If the patient has been using assistive devices for a long period of time before the amputation, or if they have used a WC or expect to use a WC for long periods of time, UE nerve function and posture should be addressed. Usually, before prosthetics, the patient is spending more time sitting and with a walker or crutches. Addressing posture of the pelvis and head/shoulders can help minimize nerve entrapment and compression. These postures do not automatically change once the patient is up and walking or have prosthetics.

Trunk and pelvic motion needed for gait, and normal motion are difficult to mimic when the patient is not ambulatory. The authors use many of the neurologic treatment including proprioceptive neuromuscular facilitation in the pelvis, trunk, and scapula to help prepare the patient for ambulation. Particularly for the bilateral and quadruple amputee, trunk strengthening can be more important than lower extremity strengthening. Pelvic and scapular posture/position should be optimized for efficiency and ease of core recruitment for all mobility and ADLs. Any patient that has spent a long time in the hospital or with an injury or illness has likely altered posture and movement patterns. The traditional sling-back WC reinforces posterior pelvic posture as well as rounded shoulders and forward head posture. Trunk and pelvic disassociation can be started with scooting transfers and bed mobility that encourages trunk rotation. Progression includes hands-on passive range of motion, active-assisted range of motion, active range of motion and resisted ROM. The authors use joint mobilization, nerve mobilization, and soft tissue mobilization in all of their patients to maximize efficient posture.

Patients who have lost their limb due to cancer comprise less than 1% of all amputees (see article by Varma and colleagues elsewhere in this issue). However, they make up a relatively large percentage of the caseload at the authors' hospital in both lower and UEs. The cancer amputee has different needs than the vascular or diabetic amputee. Cancer-related fatigue has been seen in greater than 80% of patients treated with radiation or chemotherapy. It can persist for years or months after cancer treatment. Not only is cancer-related fatigue one of the most common symptoms, it is also widely reported by patients as having the most impact on ADLs and one of the most distressing. It has a significant impact on employment and financial status.[24] Amputees require increased energy to perform ADLs and work as well as have more stress on their remaining joints.[8] Cancer treatment is also associated with neuropathy and myopathy. The cancer amputee often has very poor core strength, particularly with hip extension and trunk stability. The return of strength has a highly variable timeframe and the patient should regularly be reevaluated.

The authors' rehabilitation team has treated several quadruple amputees from a critical illness and multiple multilimb amputees from trauma, such as high-voltage electric burn. These patients can present with significant muscle weakness and neuropathy. This weakness has often been attributed to deconditioning, but may be related to critical illness neuropathy and critical illness myopathy. According to this review, the incidence of these conditions is not known, but may be up to 50% of patients in the intensive care unit with various levels of involvement.[25] The patient may present with milder findings that do not lead to extensive testing by the medical team. These very ill patients have difficulty with the demands of bed mobility and transfers following amputation that seem excessive and longer lasting than just deconditioning would account for. The authors quadruple amputee caseload from sepsis is very small, and conclusions cannot be made until there is further study. The authors have seen poor scapular stability and core/glut strength in the quadruple amputees that lasts for months and even up to a year in the face of intensive rehabilitation. Any patient who has been hospitalized for a long period of time should be continuously re-evaluated for progress and monitored to avoid rotator cuff injury or low back injury.

The authors' rehabilitation program spends time addressing safety concerns in emergency situations and includes family members. A plan should be in place for escape of the home in a hurry. The authors work on floor transfers and can spend time on crawling or hopping if it is a needed skill. Home evaluations often occur during the rehabilitation hospital stay and should be considered early for the multilimb patient as well as the patient with multiple comorbidities.

The authors also work with care providers to ensure that transfers are safe for the patient and family. If family is assisting in the care of the patient at home, the authors review the safety and technique that is used. For example, the 6-foot, 3-inch TFA husband who needs help transferring is concerned about his 5-foot, 2-inch wife who had back surgery and has a heart condition. Transfer training, education, and communication of expectations are vital to success at home. The therapists are often the health care provider that spends the most time with the patient and family and is in a great position to help start a dialogue with the other care providers. The amount of ADL assistance can also change over time. The authors meet with the psychologist in the team meetings to facilitate communication of needs from both the patient and the caregiver.

The postoperative amputee has many potential sources of pain after surgery. The therapist needs to be diligent to determine and treat pain. The patient and the medical team need to have the same vocabulary to discuss pain and determine if the pain is phantom limb pain, residual limb pain, mechanical pain, nerve pain, or phantom sensation. In the case of phantom pain, it can be difficult to rule out lumbar or even cervical dysfunction that could create radicular pain (refer to the by Uustal and Meier elsewhere in this issue).

The authors teach their unilateral patients mirror therapy. There have been case studies in the literature, but no high-quality studies demonstrating that it is effective.[19] The authors have found that it can help some patients. A few clinic aspects that the authors have found helpful in their population follow: the patient needs to be walked through the technique more than once; instructions need to be clear and concise. The mirror needs to be large enough and placed so that the residual limb is not visible; the patient should move the sound limb only at the same speed, direction, and amount the phantom limb can move. The amount of motion can increase with practice. The technique should be completed at least 5 times a week for 10 to 15 minutes once a day (**Fig. 6**).

There are other pain modalities as well. The authors have used transcutaneous electrical nerve stimulation, ice, heat, soft tissue mobilization, mobilizations, and Associate Awareness Technique with limited success.

For UE amputees, as outlined above, OT and PT see all amputees. The PT evaluation of the UE amputee involves assessment of posture, endurance, core and scapular strength, foot skills, balance, and lower extremity mobility.

Unilateral UE amputees are prone to have musculoskeletal pain in the neck/upper back, shoulders, and the sound limb.[26] They are more prone to cumulative trauma

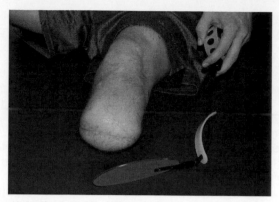

Fig. 6. A demonstration of mirror therapy.

disorders. A high percentage of unilateral UE amputees reported bilateral arm pain and that use of a prosthesis does not necessarily prevent pain.[19] The authors' experience has been that UE amputees have a tendency of elevating the scapula of the involved limb, leaning the trunk to the amputated side and flexing the lower cervical spine. The higher the amputation, usually the more pronounced the postural changes are. Maximizing mobility and stability of all of the remaining joints is a goal of the authors' rehabilitation program. The authors use PT to mobilize the soft tissue and joints in the trunk, pelvis, and scapula to improve posture and ROM. Trunk stability will also allow them to use the remaining limbs more efficiently.

The most vital participation in the whole process is the amputee's participation. The authors have often had disagreements with the patient in prioritizing skills and activities. For example, with one quadruple amputee, the authors thought that independence in toileting was the team's early priority. For the patient, his top priority was to modify his game controller so that he could return to his Internet gaming. Internet gaming allowed him to return to some of his normal social interaction. The authors cannot ignore his goal and expect him to follow their program. Socialization is a very large concern for many amputees young and old. If they see the team persuing their priorities, they are more likely to be actively involved in their treatment plan. Rehabilitation sessions may be a compromise, but the authors get more out of active participants that bring their perspective to the table than those that do not. The authors have learned something from each patient they have treated and still have more to learn.

REFERENCES

1. Hunter J, Schneider LH, Mackin E, et al. Rehabilitation of the hand: surgery and therapy. St. Louis, Missouri: C. V. Mosby CO; 1990.
2. Meier R, Atkins D. Functional restoration of adult and children with upper extremity amputation. New York: Demos Medical Publishing; 2004.
3. Finsen V, Persen L, Løvlien M, et al. Transcutaneous electrical nerve stimulation after major amputation. J Bone Joint Surg Br 1988;70(1):109–12.
4. Kim SY, Kim YY. Mirror therapy for phantom limb pain. Korean J Pain 2012;25(4): 272–4. http://dx.doi.org/10.3344/kjp.2012.25.4.272.
5. Subedi B, Grossberg GT. Phantom limb pain: mechanisms and treatment approaches. Pain Res Treat 2011;2011:864605. http://dx.doi.org/10.1155/2011/864605.

6. Robbins JM, Strauss G, Aron D, et al. Mortality rates and diabetic foot ulcers: is it time to communicate the mortality risk to the patient with diabetic foot ulceration? J Am Podiatr Med Assoc 2008;98(6):489–93.

7. Stineman MG, Kwong PL, Kurichi JE, et al. The effectiveness of inpatient rehabilitation in the acute postoperative phase of care after transtibial or transfemoral amputation: study of an integrated health care delivery system. Arch Phys Med Rehabil 2008;89(10):1863–72.

8. Iraj B, Khorvash F, Ebneshahidi A, et al. Prevention of diabetic foot ulcer. Int J Prev Med 2013;4(3):373–6.

9. O'Sullivan S, Schmitz T. Physical rehabilitation. 5th edition. Philadelphia: FA Davis Company; 2007.

10. Papazafiropoulou A, Tentolouris N, Soldatos RP, et al. Mortality in diabetic and nondiabetic paytients after amputations performed from 1196-2005 in a tertiary hospital population: a 3 year follow-up study. J Diabetes Complications 2009; 23(1):7–11.

11. Smith D. Postoperative dressing and management strategies for transtibial amputations: a critical review. J Rehabil Res Dev 2003;40(3):213–24.

12. Huang S, Ferris DP. Muscle activation patterns during walking form the transtibial amputees recorded within the residual limb-prosthetic interface. J Neuroeng Rehabil 2012;9:55.

13. Seyedali M, Czerniecki JM, Morgenroth DC, et al. Co-contraction patterns of trans-tibial amputee ankle and knee musculature during gait. J Neuroeng Rehabil 2012;9:29.

14. Dionne CP, Ertl JJW, Day JD. Rehabilitation for those with transtibial osteomyoplastic amputation. J Prosthet Orthot 2009;21(1):64–70.

15. Kegek B, Burgess EM, Starr TW, et al. Effects of isometric muscle training on residual limb volume and gait of below knee amputees. Phys Ther 1981;61(10):1419–26.

16. Nashitz, Lenger R. Why traumatic leg amputees are at increased risk for cardiovascular diseases. QJM 2008;101(4):251–9.

17. Magalhães P, Capingana DP, Silva AB, et al. Arterial stiffness in lower limb amputees. Clin Med Insights Circ Respir Pulm Med 2011;5:48–56.

18. Moseley, Gallace A, Spence C. Is mirror therapy all it is cracked up to be? Current evidence and future directions. Pain 2008;138:7–10.

19. Gailey R, Allen K, Castles J, et al. Review of secondary physical conditions associated with lower-limb amputation and long-term prosthetic use. J Rehabil Res Dev 2008;45(1):15–30.

20. Sansam K, O'Connor RJ, Neumann V, et al. Can simple clinic tests predict walking ability after prosthetic rehabilitation. J Rehabil Med 2012;44:968–74.

21. Nolan L. A training programme to improve hip strength in persons with lower limb amputation. J Rehabil Med 2012;44:241–8.

22. Soares AS, Yamaguti EY, Mochizuki L, et al. Biomechanical parameters of gait among transtibial amputees: a review. Sao Paulo Med J 2009;27(5):302–9.

23. Pyo J, Pasquina PF, Demarco M, et al. Upper limb nerve entrapment syndroms in veterans with lower limb amputations. PM R 2010;2(1):14–22.

24. Hofman M, Ryan JL, Figueroa-Moseley CD, et al. Cancer-related fatigue: the scale of the problem. Oncologist 2007;12(Suppl 1):4–10.

25. Chawla J, Davidson DL, Brasha-Mitchell E, et al. Management of critical illness polyneuropathy and myopathy. Neurol Clin 2010;28:961–77.

26. Ostiie K, Franklin RJ, Skjeldal OH, et al. Musculoskeletal pain and overuse syndrome in adult acquired major upper-limb amputees. Arch Phys Med Rehabil 2011;92:1967–73.

Prosthetic Choices for People with Leg and Arm Amputations

Robert S. Kistenberg, MPH, L/CP

KEYWORDS

• Prosthetics • Amputation • Artificial limbs • Amputees

KEY POINTS

• Provision of a prosthesis is only a component of prosthetic rehabilitation. It takes a coordinated team to optimize outcomes and functional independence.
• The most sophisticated components are not the most appropriate for everyone. All options must be weighed with consideration of the person who will be wearing the prosthesis, their environment, and *realistic* goals.
• Suspension is integral in most socket designs and must be optimized in order to prevent rubbing, slipping and fitting complications.

INTRODUCTION

Prosthesis (*noun*): a single artificial limb

Prostheses (*plural noun*): more than one artificial limb

Prosthetic (*adjective*): of or relating to artificial limbs (ie, prosthetic leg)

Prosthetics (*noun*): the profession or field of study related to artificial limbs

The explosion of options that modern technology has afforded individuals who sustain amputations or who are born with congenital limb deficiencies can be overwhelming for health care practitioners and people who rely on prosthetic technology alike. Powered, microprocessor-equipped components offer enhanced control and sophistication. Material and technology advances, improved socket designs, surgical techniques, and prosthetic rehabilitation have empowered prosthetists (and the health care team) with the ability to truly deliver the most advanced prostheses ever invented. This trend will continue in perpetuity.

Yet the most sophisticated device is not the most appropriate for everyone. The excitement provided through the media often gives people unrealistic expectations

Georgia Institute of Technology, School of Applied Physiology, 555 14th Street, Atlanta, GA 30318, USA
E-mail address: robcp@gatech.edu

Phys Med Rehabil Clin N Am 25 (2014) 93–115
http://dx.doi.org/10.1016/j.pmr.2013.10.001
1047-9651/14/$ – see front matter © 2014 Elsevier Inc. All rights reserved.

of the capacities that can be attained through the utilization of the latest and greatest. And for people who are not candidates for the best currently available prostheses, for what type of prostheses *are* they candidates? Strong scientific evidence dictating choices regarding specific components, suspension systems, and/or socket designs does not (yet) exist. How do you choose?

The aim of this article is to present the options that are available for people who rely on artificial limbs to enhance their quality of life for mobility and independence. Components by name, manufacturer, or coding category have been bypassed in lieu of a focus on features and considerations that must be made in order to make informed decisions; however, specific examples are included. Sockets, liners, and suspension systems for all levels of amputation or limb deficiency are presented first, followed by sections about feet, ankles, knees, and hip joints (for lower limb prostheses) and then sections on terminal devices, wrists, elbows, and shoulder joints (for upper limb prostheses). Although funding sources play a significant and often primary role in decisions regarding access to prosthetic rehabilitation services, the impact of funding limitations on one's choices related to prosthetic rehabilitation services are not considerations of this article.

SOCKETS, LINERS, AND SUSPENSION SYSTEMS

> If the interface between the wearer and the device is intolerable, nothing else matters.

Contemporary socket designs include lightweight carbon outer frames wrapped thoughtfully around advanced thermoplastic, anatomically optimized shells. Socket liner technology has evolved from wool socks and polyethylene foam to liners made from urethane, silicones, or thermoplastic elastomers. Grouped generically as *gel* liners, they are the most commonly used prosthetic interface in North America. All gel-type liners must be rolled onto a residual limb with careful attention to avoid air between the skin and the liner; hence, dexterity is required for independent donning. Liners also require daily washing, require regular replacement (6–12 months), may be hot, and perceived as bulky. Different types of liners are integral to different suspension systems.

Cushion liners consist of different thicknesses of gel with or without a fabric covering and are rarely sufficient to provide suspension alone (**Fig. 1**). In transtibial applications, they are combined with a knee sleeve, which seals the residual limb/socket chamber, and an expulsion valve creating a suction socket. The chamber is created between the inner surface of the prosthetic socket and the outer surface of the liner, not between the liner and the skin. Negative pressure (subatmospheric) is created when the residual limb is pressed into the socket on loading and subsequently extracted during unloading. Variations of this sealed suction system have been used on transfemoral, hip disarticulation, and upper limb prostheses.

Elevated vacuum (also known as vacuum assisted) suspension takes the same system described earlier; however, the negative pressure in the chamber is increased by the addition of an electric or mechanical vacuum pump. Elevated vacuum suspension reduces residual limb pistoning,[1] reduces residual limb volume loss,[1–4] and has demonstrated value in residual limb wound healing.[5] In addition to added weight and the need for daily charging (for electric pump systems), the knee sleeve may restrict the knee range of motion in transtibial elevated vacuum wearers. Liners for

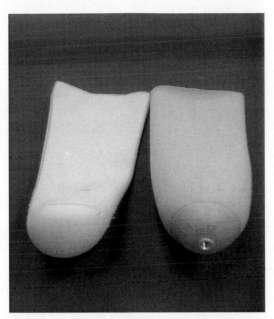

Fig. 1. Cushion liner is on the left, and locking liner is on the right.

an elevated vacuum are most often made of urethane or silicone. If the knee sleeve is punctured, the suspension is compromised.

To provide the benefits of a sealed chamber suspension while eliminating the proximal sleeve, some cushion liners have one or more sealing rings on their outer surface that press against the socket inner wall to create the atmospheric chamber (**Fig. 2**). Liners with sealing rings can be used with expulsion valves or elevated vacuum suspension.

Locking liners are cushion liners with an umbrella-shaped threaded nut at the distal end into which pins, straps, or lanyards are installed. These distal attachments, in turn, are secured to the exterior of the socket (using straps and lanyards) or to distal shuttle locks (pins) to provide a mechanically locked attachment between the liner and the prosthesis (**Fig. 3**) As locking liner suspensions concentrate the suspension force at the distal end of the socket, they may create a milking effect on the distal residual limb in people with lower limb amputations.

Atmospheric Suspension, Anatomic Suspension, and Osseointegration

Movement between the residual limb and the prosthesis, or the lack thereof, is determined by the prosthetic suspension system. Any suspension system that relies on an air chamber being created to prevent or minimize prosthetic slippage can be categorized as atmospheric suspension. Skin fit suction suspension, knee sleeves, liner-assisted pin and lanyard systems, and elevated vacuum are all types of atmospheric suspension systems. An alternative to atmospheric suspension systems is anatomic suspension.

Anatomic suspension consists of hanging a prosthesis over a boney prominence. This technique can be achieved by having wedges or bladders built into a prosthetic socket or by using strapping and belts. When atmospheric suspensions are not feasible, anatomic suspension systems often provide a solution. It is not uncommon for a single prosthesis to have more than one type of suspension mechanism. For

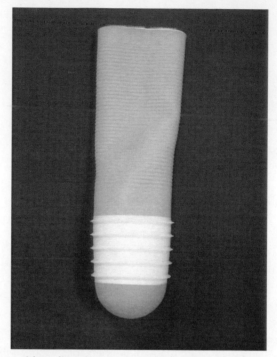

Fig. 2. Cushion liner with sealing rings.

people that have serious socket-fitting and/or suspension challenges, osseointegration presents as another promising solution.

Available in Europe, osseointegration is the ultimate prosthetic suspension system because it eliminates the need for a socket altogether by attaching the prosthetic components directly to a skeletally integrated implant. Surgical procedures and healing time are necessary for the implant to become integrated before prosthetic fitting can commence. Ease of donning, decreased energy expenditure, and improved hip range of motion have been reported in people with osseointegrated transfemoral amputations.[6] Transfemoral is the most common level for osseointegration; however, it

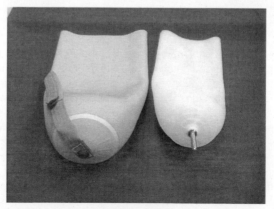

Fig. 3. Locking liners with straps (*right*) and pin (*left*).

has also been successfully applied to transtibial, digital, transradial, and transhumeral level amputations. The incidence of infection is one of the reasons osseointegration has not received approval by the Food and Drug Administration in the United States; however, human trials are undergoing.[7]

LOWER LIMB PROSTHETICS
Prosthetic Foot and Ankle Mechanisms

Prosthetic feet are often grouped according to historical categories because these categories evolved to become descriptors for reimbursement codes. Examples of common foot categories include solid ankle cushion heel (SACH) feet, flexible keel feet, dynamic response feet, and single axis and multi axis feet; however, it has been acknowledged that the codes (categories) into which feet have been assigned lack a standardized methodology to test mechanical abilities.[8] Scientific evidence to recommend specific prosthetic foot-ankle mechanisms is lacking.[9] As early as 1975, Daher[10] demonstrated that even feet within the same category do not perform the same in mechanical testing. Rather than using historical categories, the following sections focus on primary prosthetic foot selection considerations, the prosthetic foot keel, the prosthetic foot heel, as well as prosthetic foot aesthetics and shoes.

Primary Foot Selection Considerations

Two foot-choice considerations are inviolate: weight rating and build height. All feet are designed to support a certain amount of load. A foot's weight rating must be considered with the wearer's body weight *plus* any loads they may eventually carry to be structurally safe. Prosthetic foot build height is the amount of space required to install a prosthetic foot such that it will fit between the ground and the distal end of the residual limb. One should not install a prosthetic foot on someone who weighs more than the foot is designed to withstand. One cannot install a prosthetic foot that requires clearance space that does not exist (**Fig. 4**).

Taken from the surgical perspective, the amount of limb amputated results in clearance space for the available prosthetic components. If one asks what the ideal amputation length for a transtibial amputation is, the answer depends on the type of foot/ankle mechanism for which the individual is indicated and how much they weigh. **Table 1** presents build heights and weight ratings for different prosthetic feet (based on representative examples).

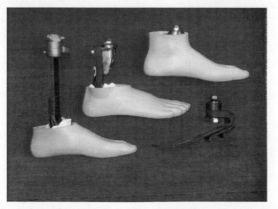

Fig. 4. Three prosthetic feet with varying build heights. The item in the bottom right corner is a foot keel without the foot shell covering.

Table 1 Carbon fiber prosthetic foot/ankle mechanisms with build height and weight ratings for amputations distal to the knee		
Foot/Ankle Type	Build Height/ Space Needed (cm)	Weight Rating (lb)
Chopart foot	.6	324
Syme level foot	6	365
Intrinsic keel carbon foot	10–12	500
Extrinsic keel carbon foot	Up to 35	440
CF running blades	19–42	365
CF with hydraulic ankle	10–12	220–275
CF with hydraulic ankle + microprocessor control	10–18	220–275
CF with hydraulic ankle + microprocessor control + active power generation	22	250

Abbreviation: CF, carbon fiber.

After abiding to the weight rating and build height limitations, subsequent prosthetic foot considerations are bound by the wearer's activity level and aesthetic preferences. The activity level defines functional demands. The extent to which a foot (or feet) can meet functional demands and aesthetic preferences is the extent to which it (or they) will be acceptable to the wearer.

> The extent to which any prosthesis (prostheses) can meet the functional demands and aesthetic preferences of the wearer delineates the boundaries of prosthetic acceptance and rejection.

The Prosthetic Foot Keel

With the exception of peg legs, the most critical component of any prosthetic foot is the keel. The keel is the part of the prosthetic foot that simulates the human musculo-skeletal anatomic structures responsible for structural stability and mobility during loading and movement. For some people with lower limb amputations, stability is paramount; for others, mobility is the primary objective. Prosthetic foot keels, historically made of hardwood, are now made using a variety of materials, such as Delrin or Kevlar (DuPont, Wilmington, DE); urethane; and, most commonly, carbon fiber composites. Some keels are split to facilitate the simulation of inversion/eversion of the prosthetic foot (**Fig. 5**).

Before the introduction of the carbon keel becoming extrinsic to the foot, prosthetic feet had keels that were intrinsic to the foot. Adding carbon and other dynamic materials to foot keels facilitated feet that first could accommodate terrain and absorb shock (ie, *flexible keel* and *multiaxial* feet) followed by feet that could store and return energy (also known as *dynamic response* or *energy storage and return* feet) and then ultimately to keels that combined features (multiaxial, dynamic response feet) and feet designed for running.

The Prosthetic Foot Heel

At the initial contact/loading response phase of the gait cycle, a prosthetic foot must simultaneously absorb shock and maintain forward progression. Human feet

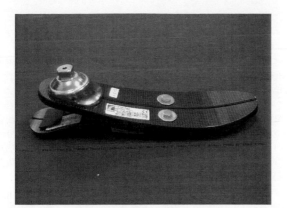

Fig. 5. Low-profile split keel foot without foot shell.

accomplish this through the evolved capacities of the fat pad of the heel, the bones and ligaments of the foot ankle complex, as well as eccentric contraction of the pre-tibial muscles of the shank. Prosthetic feet accomplish shock absorption and mainte-nance of forward momentum in several ways, the simplest is the cushioned foam heels or interchangeable foam heel plugs. Single and multiaxial feet use elastic bumpers that prosthetists tune to the wearer's gait. In some instances, the heel durometer can be adjustable by the wearer.

Having a prosthetic foot that plantarflexes, either through articulation (single and multiaxial feet) or simulation (cushioned heels or keel deformation), reduces the knee flexion moment for the wearer in the early stance, which ultimately increases knee stability. This stability is vital for people with transtibial amputations with compro-mised knee extensors and for people with transfemoral amputations who have a compromised ability to control the prosthetic knee.

Aesthetics of Prosthetic Feet and Shoes

Historically, foot appearance and even color were considered unimportant because feet were always meant to be worn in a shoe. As the foot-manufacturing processes improved, feet of varying skin shades and sculpted features became available. With the expansion of carbon fiber feet came the introduction of the foot shell, which not only mimics human foot appearance but it also protects the carbon composite keel. Foot shells and prosthetic feet with intrinsic keels come in different skin tones and levels of detail. A split toe option between the great and second toes facilitates wearing san-dals and flip-flops. Sculpted toes and toenails allow for polish to be added if desired.

Apart from prosthetic foot-ankle mechanisms with microprocessors that automati-cally adjust to the heel height of the shoe, prosthetic feet are designed to be worn with shoes that have a specific heel height. Wearing shoes with heel heights that differ from the shoes with which the prosthesis was initially aligned without accommodating for the heel height differences will adversely affect the performance of the foot, potentially causing injury to the residual limb and/or increasing risk for falls. To facilitate wearing shoes with different heel heights, feet with user-adjustable heel heights are available.

Prosthetic Ankles and Shanks

In general, motions attributable to human ankles are incorporated into prosthetic foot designs; therefore, separate ankle components are often unnecessary. Exceptions are when vertical loading and/or torsional demands go beyond the capabilities of the prosthetic foot (for example, with golf or basketball). To meet these demands, vertical shock pylons and torque absorbers are available.

Although the application of hydraulics to dampen ankle motion is not new,[11] several manufacturers have recently reintroduced hydraulically controlled ankle mechanisms as a means to passively adapt to different terrains. The addition of microprocessors to prosthetic foot/ankle mechanisms to control ankle motion allows prosthetic feet to behave similarly to human feet. For example, the prosthetic foot/ankle mechanism can dorsiflex during the swing phase to facilitate toe clearance and automatically adapt to different heel heights between shoes. The recent introduction of an actively powered prosthetic foot/ankle mechanism (BiOM Ankle System, iWalk Inc, Bedford, MA) now allows for gait performance of people with lower limb amputations to not be statistically significantly different from that of people without amputations across different gait velocities.[12] The downside to the addition of these sophisticated components is the added weight, bulk, maintenance, and financial cost.

Prosthetic Knees

Prosthetic knees and the ability to control them have a drastic effect on the quality of life for individuals with knee disarticulations or more proximal lower limb amputation levels. People with amputations who lack the ability to maintain the prosthetic knee in extension during the stance phase or insufficient flexion during the swing phase for toe clearance are at risk for falls. Active community ambulators who vary their cadence and terrain require a knee that can accommodate ever-changing speeds and conditions. Before the advent of microprocessor control of prosthetic knees, wearers would often comment that they had to think about every step in order to prevent inadvertent knee collapse and falls. When compared with walking with non–microprocessor-controlled knees, people report that walking requires less attention when wearing a microprocessor-controlled knee (MPKs).[13]

The impact that microprocessor control has had on prosthetic knees is so significant that knees are now categorized as either exclusive mechanical control (non-MPKs) or MPKs.[14] By way of introduction to knee designs and features, the following sections on knee axis configurations, fluid dampening versus constant friction, and 4 additional knee features are specific to non-MPKs. The subsequent section addresses MPKs.

Knee Axis Configurations

Historically, prosthetic knees were categorized according to their axis design (single axis vs polycentric knees) because different axis designs were indicated based on the wearer's residual limb length, functional demands, and their ability to control the knee. For non-MPKs, these indications still apply. As the name implies, single-axis knees rotate about one axis and are mechanically simpler and lighter than their polycentric counterparts.

Polycentric knees (also known as 4-bar knees, although some designs have greater than 4 linkages) actually rotate around an infinite number of axes as an *instantaneous center of rotation* changes as the knee flexes or extends (**Fig. 6**). The advantages of polycentric knees include inherent stance stability, shortening in the swing phase, and a low build height (critical for long transfemoral and knee disarticulation amputations when sitting).[15]

Fluid Dampening Versus Constant Friction

The difference between using a prosthetic knee with constant friction or with fluid dampening relates to the wearer's ability or inability to ambulate at different speeds.

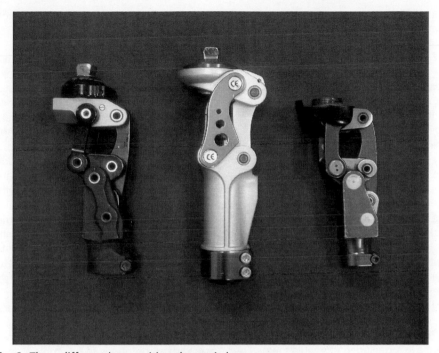

Fig. 6. Three different knees with polycentric knee axes.

Single-speed walkers are generally household or limited community ambulators and do not need a prosthetic knee that is responsive to changing speeds. Hence, they are indicated for knees with constant friction as it relates to knee flexion/extension. The amount of friction can be adjusted by the prosthetist; however, once set, it remains constant.

Individuals who ambulate with variable cadence are indicated for prosthetic knees with fluid dampening. Depending on the functional demands, the fluid may be hydraulic, pneumatic, or, in some instances, both. Fluid motion dampening may occur in the swing phase only, stance phase only, or both swing and stance phases of the gait. Adjustments to fluid dampening are expressed in terms of resistance to motion. For example, a prosthetist would increase resistance to knee flexion motion if excessive heel rise was observed in the initial swing phase of the gait. Resistance to knee flexion adjustments and resistance to knee extension adjustments are performed independently of one another. Resistance to flexion/extension in stance adjustments is performed independent of resistance adjustments in the swing.

Four Additional Knee Features

In response to the critical need for knee control in conjunction with inherent limitations resulting from high-level lower limb amputations, 4 additional knee features exist that aid in knee stability and/or improve gait. These features are (1) manual locks, (2) extension assists, (3) weight-activated stance control, and (4) stance flexion. Depending on the functional demands for which a prosthetic knee is designed, it may have none, one, or some combination of these features.

People indicated for knees with *manual locks* are either very-low-level household ambulators or have a functional demand requiring the prosthetic knee locked for an extended period of time (for example, when one's job requires them to stand in one place). The lock is disengaged for sitting; however, this requires hand dexterity, which may be a challenge for those who require an assistive device, such as a walker, for stability.

Extension assists are elastic components that facilitate the prosthetic knee to attain full extension once it has flexed during the swing phase. People with general weakness or with weak hip flexors are indicated for knees that have extension assists. Extension assists are adjustable because excessive assistance can result in the prosthetic knee snapping into full extension with an audible terminal impact. Prosthetists adjust extension-assist components in harmony with constant friction or fluid dampening adjustments because these aspects of prosthetic knee function are interrelated.

Weight-activated stance control is a feature that uses a braking mechanism to lock the knee if weight is applied while the knee is not in full extension. Individuals who are low-level walkers or identified with a fall risk are indicated for a prosthetic knee with weight-activated stance control. The amount of weight required to activate the brake is adjustable, and different knees offer different ranges of knee flexion within which the weight-activated stance control will engage. To induce knee flexion for a knee with weight-activated stance control, it needs to be fully unweighted. This may result in awkward transitions from the preswing to the initial swing phase of the gait. It also may present challenges for initiating flexion when sitting. Although weight-activated stance control is a safety feature of prosthetic knees, exercise caution when referring to this type of knee as a *safety* knee because this is misleading and may open practitioners up to liability.

The fourth feature for prosthetic knees, *stance flexion*, differs from the first 3 because it is designed to enable the gait of people with amputations to resemble a non-amputated gait by allowing for some amount of knee flexion at the initial contact/loading response phases of walking. Although initially posited by Saunders and colleagues[16] to play a role in reducing vertical trunk displacement, stance-phase knee flexion was determined by Gard and Childress[17] to play a role not in vertical displacement but in shock absorption. Attenuating shock for people with transfemoral amputations is vital because chronic low-back pain has been documented in people with lower extremity amputations.[18,19] Hence, the stance flexion feature in prosthetic knees is appropriate for individuals who are variable-cadence community ambulators and/or at risk for back pain. It should be noted that the transition from a prosthetic knee without stance flexion to a knee with stance flexion may be challenging because the sensation of knee bending at initial contact/loading response is associated with knee buckling and falling by people accustomed to knees without stance flexion.

Every prosthetic knee, either non-MPK or MPK, will have either a single axis or polycentric design; every prosthetic knee requires some method to control its motion. The 4 additional features described earlier for non-MPKs may or may not be present depending on the population for which a particular knee was designed. The introduction of microprocessors to prosthetic knees has allowed prosthetic designs to incorporate the aforementioned features either through mechanical means, microprocessor control, or a combination of both.

Microprocessor Control of Prosthetic Knees

The first prosthetic knee to incorporate microprocessor control of the swing phase was the Blatchford Intelligent Prosthesis (IP, Chas A Blatchford & Sons Ltd, Hampshire, United Kingdom) in the early 1990s.[14] The C-Leg (Ottobock, Duderstadt, Germany), introduced in the late 1990s, was the first prosthetic knee with microprocessor control of both the swing and stance phase. Although intelligent swing-phase control may optimize the swing, microprocessor stance-phase control is the feature that launched the MPK revolution. With stance control, the prosthetic knee could respond automatically to varying conditions of stair and ramp ascent and descent as well as uneven terrains, conditions exceptionally challenging for most people with high-level lower limb amputations.

The introduction of the Power Knee (Össur, Reykjavik, Iceland) in 2006 brought microprocessor control of the prosthetic knee to the next level by not only controlling the knee's motion but also by actively adding power to the knee, reportedly facilitating the ability for people with transfemoral amputations to walk up stairs step over step. Comparing the Power Knee with the C-Leg in stair and ramp ascent and descent among 5 young and motivated people with unilateral transfemoral amputations, Wolf and colleagues[20] concluded that the Power Knee did significantly reduce the power generated by the nondisabled knee during stair ascent as designed. Wolf and colleagues[21] also compared the 2 knees for sit-to-stand and step-up tasks and found no significant differences between either of the affected limbs or the intact limb when comparing devices. The latest innovation with regard to lower limb prosthetics is the incorporation of a MPK and foot working in harmony as is seen in the Symbionic leg (Össur, Reykjavik, Iceland).

Although the advantages of microprocessor control have been well publicized, before choosing a MCK one must also consider the need for regular charging, moisture restrictions, added weight, and the short- and long-term costs.

Transverse Rotators: an Important Component for People with Transfemoral Amputations

For individuals who have transfemoral amputations and who have enough clearance between the end of their residual limb and their prosthetic knee joint, the addition of a transverse rotator can make the difference between acceptance and rejection of a prosthesis. With the push of a button, the section of the prosthesis distal to the socket can freely rotate in the transverse plane. This function enables the wearer to change their shoes without forward flexing at the waist or having to remove their prosthesis. Transverse rotators can facilitate getting into a vehicle and comfortable sitting in a vehicle. For individuals who sit on the floor, they allow one to sit with their legs crossed. Once the rotator is placed back in its proper alignment, it locks into place.

Transverse rotation adapters add less than 1 in of component build height between the top of the prosthetic knee joint and the bottom of the prosthetic socket, add less than 200 g to the weight of the prosthesis, and are weight rated for individuals who weigh up to 330 lb.

Prosthetic Hip Joints

Hip disarticulation, hemipelvectomy, and some very short transfemoral amputations require a prosthetic hip joint to restore anatomic functions. Because this level of amputation is rare compared with more distal lower limb amputations, component options are limited. The prosthetic hip joint must remain stable throughout the stance phase and facilitate limb clearance and knee joint flexion through the swing phase. In addition, it should allow for comfortable level sitting. Conventional hip joints consist of a single axis joint with adjustability for alignment in the transverse and sagittal plane. Because the market for hip joints is rather limited, new hip joints are uncommon. An exception is the Helix3D hip joint (Ottobock, Duderstadt, Germany) introduced in 2008.

The Helix3D hip joint incorporates a novel polycentric design as well as hydraulics for both swing- and stance-phase control (**Fig. 7**). Recognizing the interdependence of the prosthetic hip and knee joint, the Helix3D system must be coupled with a compatible C-Leg or Genium (Ottobock, Duderstadt, Germany) knee in order to function properly.

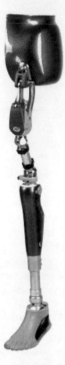

Fig. 7. Hip disarticulation prosthesis with helix3D system. (*Courtesy of* Ottobock, Duder-stadt, Germany; with permission.)

In a single case study following a 30-year-old male veteran with a hip disarticulation amputation over 15 weeks, Nelson and Carbone[22] documented that while using the Helix3D system, the patient was able to ambulate at a speed indicating independence in activities of daily living and successful community ambulation; he was not able to obtain the same level of ambulation with the conventional single-axis hip joint.

Summary of Options for People with Lower Limb Amputations

The aforementioned sections provide a snapshot of the available components and features thereof for individuals who sustain lower limb amputations and are indicated for a prosthetic rehabilitation. Although not exhaustive, this section focuses on the de-velopments about which health care practitioners ought to be informed. The same approach is used for the following section on upper limb prosthetics.

UPPER LIMB PROSTHETICS

> No one upper limb prosthesis will replace the innumerable functions of the human arm and hand.

Individuals with upper limb amputations have different choices than people with lower limb amputations because people do infinitely more with their hands than with their feet. Upper limb prostheses do not restore the lost functions of the arms to the extent that lower limb prostheses do for legs. Choosing not to wear a lower limb prosthesis leaves one with the options of wheelchair ambulation, hopping with a walker or a swing-through gait on crutches. One's quality of life, mobility, and independence is definitely impacted.

For unilateral upper limb amputations, choosing not to wear a prosthesis leaves one one-handed in a two-handed world but may have minimal to no effect on mobility or independence. The effect of an upper limb amputation on one's quality of life, however, is as varied as the people who have upper limb amputations. A concert pianist has a finger amputated and he or she is devastated. Another person may display his or her lost finger as a badge of courage.

The emphasis for prosthetic rehabilitation for people with upper limb amputations should be that a prosthesis is a tool to facilitate goal attainment and that different designs may be necessary to achieve different goals. Put another way, no one upper limb prosthesis will replace the innumerable functions of the human arm and hand. Multiple terminal devices and/or multiple prostheses may be required. If an individual's prosthetic rehabilitation plan is designed to facilitate realistic goals and a prosthesis enables them to achieve those goals, rejection should only occur when one's goals have changed. Unstated or poorly defined goals are a direct path to prosthetic rejection. Furthermore, the role of occupational therapy cannot be overemphasized when it comes to upper limb prosthetic rehabilitation.

The following sections introduce different styles of prostheses (functional aesthetic and activity specific), strategies for control (body powered vs externally powered), and options for people with upper limb amputations at different levels of amputation.

Functional Aesthetic Prostheses

Often people with new upper limb amputations feel awkward in social situations because they struggle to incorporate their new physical appearance into their self-image. Provision of an aesthetic restoration for either a finger or a complete arm will *allow people with amputations to perform the illusion* that they have not had an amputation by restoring a normal appearance. It should be emphasized that this type of prosthesis is aesthetic (referring to natural beauty) rather than cosmetic (referring to not substantive or superficial). This type of prosthesis may serve as a means to facilitate acceptance and return to a premorbid social life. They may be used full time or only on occasion.

If one becomes socially reclusive as a result of their amputation or outward appearance and provision of a prosthesis facilitates the return to social engagement, that prosthesis has served an extraordinarily valuable function. Another functional benefit of aesthetic prostheses is that, although they may not be actively prehensile, they do restore the ability to perform bimanual activities for those with unilateral amputations. For people with finger amputations, silicone aesthetic finger prostheses fill a void left by the amputated digits, allowing secure grasp of small items, such as coins. People with amputations at the wrist or higher can use a functional aesthetic prosthesis to hold objects by placing them into a prepositioned hand or by wedging items between the prosthesis and the wearer's torso.

Operation of functional aesthetic prostheses is achieved through manipulation by the sound hand. For example, functional aesthetic hands have wired fingers that can be prepositioned to hold an object (**Fig. 8**). Aesthetic restoration for someone with a transhumeral amputation has an elbow that can be locked in varying degrees of flexion to allow for hanging purses or bags.

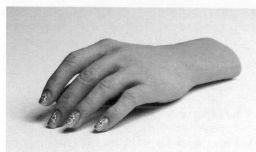

Fig. 8. Custom-sculpted silicone hand. (*Courtesy of* Touch Bionics, Mansfield, MA; with permission.)

Activity-Specific Prostheses

Sports and recreation are a significant part of people's lives, and losing the ability to participate in these activities secondary to an amputation can be dually devastating. First, an experience with friends in a social activity is lost. Second, a physical activity is eliminated. Returning to a favorite sport or recreational activity is a motivating goal for many. Fortunately, prosthetic options exist that can enable the return to an array of sport and recreational activities (**Fig. 9**). These devices, however, may not be appropriate for everyday functional tasks. An arm designed for swimming will not perform the functions necessary for office work, manual labor, or meal preparation. In some instances, a prosthesis can be made multipurpose by using a quick disconnect wrist unit and an assortment of different terminal devices. Depending on the activities and goals of the wearer, multiple prostheses may be indicated; however, many people reject the notion of having to carry around a bag of arms or extra attachments.

Strategies for Control of Upper Limb Prosthetics

Control of an upper limb prosthesis refers to the manner by which the wearer operates the various components. *Body-powered (BP)* components are those that use a harness and cabling to capture a body motion and transmit that motion into activation of a component. They tend to be more rugged, lighter weight, and less costly than *externally powered* (EP) components. *EP* components are those that have motors, batteries, microprocessors, and an input method by which the wearer can communicate their intention to the device. The input method of choice for most EP prosthesis

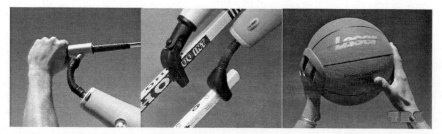

Fig. 9. Sports and recreational terminal devices. (*Courtesy of* Therapeutic Recreation Systems, Boulder, CO; with permission.)

wearers is surface electrodes. Because these electrodes use electromyography (EMG) signals, EP prostheses are also referred to as *myoelectric* prostheses; however, not all EP prostheses are myoelectric because other input types are available. For people who require independent control of multiple components, for example, an elbow, wrist, and hand, *hybrid-powered* prostheses use a combination of EP and BP. The terminal device may be EP, whereas the elbow may be BP.

Taken together, functional-aesthetic, activity-specific, BP, EP, and hybrid-powered prostheses compose the 5 prosthetic options available for people with upper limb amputations. A sixth option is to choose not to wear a prosthesis at all. The following sections detail options available according to amputation level.

Options for Thumb, Finger, and Partial Hand Amputations

> One's response to having an amputation is in no way proportional to the amount of amputation they sustain.

Historically, finger and partial hand amputations have been disregarded because prosthetic options have been few due to space limitations. Functional aesthetic options are available for people with finger and partial hand amputations. Both BP and EP prosthetic options exist for people with partial hand amputations.

Because the thumb and fingers compose 90% of human arm function,[23] the loss of one or more fingers has an effect on hand function. Custom-sculpted, hand-painted silicone digits not only restore a realistic appearance but they also offer compression and desensitization for residual fingers. These aesthetic restorations facilitate grasp by providing a textured, high-friction surface. Special considerations need to be made for thumb amputations because opposition is either diminished or lost. In some cases, an opposition post will facilitate grasp with the remaining digits.

BP options for digital and partial hand amputations attempt to harness either metacarpophalangeal or wrist flexion/extension to drive prosthetic digits. Grip force is limited to the strength attainable by these motions. Aesthetics for these types of prostheses may be sacrificed in lieu of function.

EP options for partial hand amputations are available for amputations of the thumb only or of 2 or more digits. External power affords firm grip strength for the partial hand prostheses. Although custom gloves can restore an aesthetic appearance to an EP partial hand prosthesis, some wearers prefer a high-tech look using carbon fiber or other textiles to display their individuality (**Fig. 10**). Because of space limitations, batteries and microprocessors are usually mounted on a wristband. Input for control is via surface electrodes or force sense resistors, which translate pressure into a signaling voltage.

As a downside to partial hand prostheses, many wearers report that they are hot and/or heavy. Some people prefer to leave their hand open because wearing a partial hand prosthesis impedes sensation of the residual hand.

Options for Upper Limb Amputations at the Wrist and Proximal

Terminal devices

The terminal device (TD) of an upper limb prosthesis is the component that is installed into the end of the arm. TDs are categorized according to their control strategy; hence,

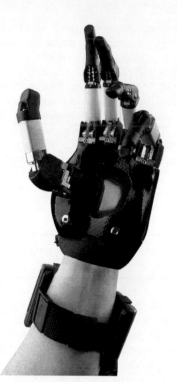

Fig. 10. EP partial hand prosthesis. (*Courtesy of* Touch Bionics, Mansfield, MA; with permission.)

they can be aesthetic, activity specific, BP, or EP. Aesthetic TDs are hands by definition. Activity-specific TDs can be tools, utensils, or any other imaginable device that facilitates the activity for which it was designed. BP and EP TDs are hands, split hooks, or prehensors.

Voluntary opening versus voluntary closing

BP TD operation is either voluntary opening (VO [pull cable to open TD]) or voluntary closing (VC [pull cable to close TD]). The pinch force for VO devices is determined by the number of rubber bands or springs installed for closure. The wearer must overcome that same amount of pinch force every time they open the TD. An advantage to VO operation is that once an object is placed into the TD and the harness/cabling relaxed, the object remains held until the TD is opened or the object is pulled out.

With VC devices, forces generated by the wearer through the cable and harness regulate the pinch force. This action creates a feedback mechanism so the wearer can learn to associate harness pressures with TD grip force. VC TDs can grip onto items being held through mechanical locks, pins, or cable cleats. When choosing a BP prosthesis, the decision between VO and VC control will dictate the availability of TD components.

Hands, split hooks, and prehensors

BP hands are designed to provide a measure of aesthetic appearance while simulating human hand cylindrical and/or 3 jaw chuck grasp patterns. To enhance appearance, they may be covered with vinyl or silicone gloves in various skin shades; however, some BP hands are aesthetically sculpted and do not require a glove. The disadvantages of BP hands are that they are visually obstructive, lack fine-tip prehension, and are comparatively heavy. BP split hooks are not visually obstructive and excel only at fine-tip prehension and lateral prehension. Hooks are lightweight and come in an array of sizes, shapes, and materials depending on the functional demands of the user. The aesthetics of a hook, however, may lead some to reject this as an option outright.

BP prehensors appear similar to split hooks, but in operation they move similar to a thumb and index finger during pinch. They are designed to facilitate grasping patterns using opposing nonidentical fingers. The motion of the prehensors' grasp facilitates cylindrical and fine-tip prehension (**Fig. 11**).

EP hands can be categorized as having nonarticulated or multiarticulated fingers. EP hands with nonarticulated fingers have one motor that drives the thumb against the second and third digits simultaneously, which creates a 3-jaw chuck grasp pattern. The fourth and fifth digits provide an aesthetic appearance but are not powered. These hands have high pinch forces between the thumb and 2 active fingers and require an outer glove for protection and aesthetics.

The iLIMB Hand (Touch Bionics, Livingston, United Kingdom), the first EP hand with multi-articulating fingers, became commercially available in 2007 (**Fig. 12**). In addition to each individual digit having a dedicated motor, the thumb mount for this multi-articulating hand allows for thumb abduction/adduction. The combination of individually powered digits and a positionable, opposable thumb facilitates hand grasping patterns and grips that closely simulated those of the human hand. Additionally, when the hand is closing (digits flexing) around an object, each digit will stop closing only when it contacts enough resistance to stall its' motor. That translates into a compliant grip similar to the way the human hand grasps objects of different shapes and sizes.

EP hands with multi-articulating fingers include microprocessors with wireless connectivity that facilitate the hand to be programed for different grasp patterns and grips in different environments (ie, work, home, or recreation). Wearers can generate triggers through the EP inputs to communicate their intention to the hand in order to change grip patterns. EP hands also require an outer glove for protection, which may be aesthetic, clear, or a variety of different colors.

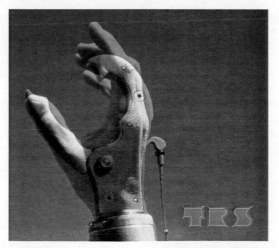

Fig. 11. Prehensor overlaid with human hand. (*Courtesy of* Therapeutic Recreation Systems, Boulder, CO; with permission.)

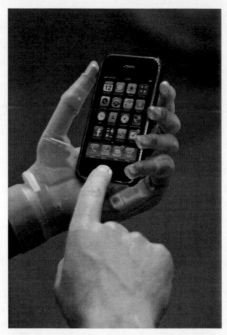

Fig. 12. EP prosthetic hand with multi-articulating fingers. (*Courtesy of* Touch Bionics, Mansfield, MA; with permission.)

EP hooks marry the visual unobstructiveness and fine-tip prehension of BP hooks with the power and control of external power. This device is often the TD of choice for BP wearers who have to transition to EP (**Fig. 13**). EP prehensors are heavy-duty vicelike devices that generate high pinch forces (160 N or almost 36 lb) and are primarily used for heavy-duty activities.

Wrists
The role of the wrist unit is to connect the TD to the rest of the prosthesis and to facilitate positioning of the TD such that compensatory motions by proximal body joints are reduced or eliminated. At a minimum, a wrist unit must offer some measure of pronation/supination in order to be functional. Some wrist units offer flexion/extension of the TD in predetermined positions. A final useful feature of the wrist unit is that of quick disconnect that allows for rapid exchange of one TD for another.

In BP wrists, pronation and supination can be accomplished manually by rotating the TD against friction or through BP activated springs and cabling. Flexion and extension motion is accessed by activation of a button or lever. Some BP wrists incorporate a ball-and-socket design that allows for universal wrist motion.

In EP wrists, the same functional demands apply; however, they are accomplished in different ways. Powered wrist rotation (pronation/supination) effectively positions the TD but its torque generation is sufficient to turn a doorknob, for example. EP wrists pronation/supination can also be accomplished by manual rotation. As with BP wrists, flexion/extension motions can be accessed by the activation of a button (**Fig. 14**); however, wrist units that offer powered flexion/extension are under development.[24] Quick disconnect of TDs for EP is also available when someone has more than one TD.

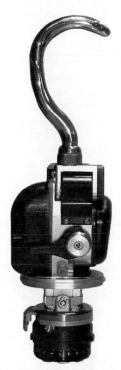

Fig. 13. EP hook TD. (*Courtesy of* Motion Control, Salt Lake City, UT; with permission.)

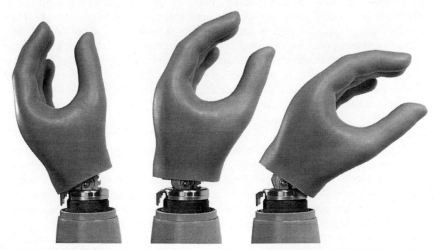

Fig. 14. EP hand on flexion extension wrist. (*Courtesy of* Motion Control, Salt lake City, UT; with permission.)

Elbows

When an amputation occurs at or above the elbow, elbow flexion and extension must be incorporated into the prosthetic design in order to facilitate TD positioning. Internal and external humeral rotation motions are achieved manually.

BP elbow joints can be positioned manually or through cable motion. Because the elbow position must remain fixed in order to maintain the terminal device in the desired location, elbow locks are also needed to prevent slippage. Elbow locks can be cable activated or manually activated. If the elbow motion is accomplished through cable activation, live lift (the amount of weight that can be held while the elbow is flexing) is limited with BP systems. In most instances with BP arms, the TD must be prepositioned with elbow flexion and wrist rotation before putting an object into the TD.

EP elbows offer powered flexion as well as powered elbow locks, each of which can be controlled through a variety of different input methods. Commonly, an input signal generates elbow flexion through its range of motion; when that signal terminates, the elbow locks. The same applies with elbow extension. As with BP elbows, humeral internal and external rotation is controlled manually. In order to operate an EP transhumeral prosthesis using only one pair of surface electrodes, the wearer would need to select and operate the elbow position, select then change the wrist position, and then ultimately select then operate the TD consecutively. This unintuitive and time-consuming process requires extensive patience, training, and determination.

Uncoupling TD activation and elbow activation by using different inputs for each allows wearers the ability to simultaneously control elbow motion and TD motion. For example, the elbow may be controlled through BP and the terminal device and wrist may be controlled through myosites. Although complex, with training and experience, fluid control of a hybrid prosthesis is possible. However, pattern recognition holds the greatest promise as a source for communicating the intent of the prosthetic wearer to their device.

Although control of a prosthetic arm through EMG pattern recognition is not new,[25,26] the development of prosthetic arms that offer comparable degrees of freedom to the human arm have fueled a pattern-recognition resurgence.[27–29] Pattern recognition is a rapidly evolving means to capture the wearer's intent for their arm prosthetic motions in an intuitive manner. First, a series of surface electrodes are placed onto their residual limb. Next, the wearer is shown a demonstration of a specific hand/wrist/arm motion and is asked to mimic that motion/muscle activation pattern to the extent possible. The resultant EMG pattern is recorded and associated with the hand/arm motion shown in the video. With repetition and practice, the system recognizes which EMG patterns are associated with which intended arm movements and directs the prosthesis to respond accordingly. Pattern recognition is also now being investigated for control of lower limb prostheses.[30,31]

Shoulders

As with hip disarticulation and hemipelvectomy amputations, shoulder disarticulation and interscapulothoracic amputations are rare, which leads to a very small market for commercial product development for people who require the greatest functional restoration. Prosthetic shoulder joints connect the socket to the remaining arm components. Versions of BP shoulder joints offer flexion/extension alone or in conjunction with abduction/adduction. These motions may be limited through constant friction or a mechanical elbow lock. Powered shoulder joints for flexion/extension are not available; however, shoulder joints with passive motion and electronic locks are available.

Options for People with Bilateral Upper Limb Amputations

People with bilateral upper limb amputations often rely on prosthetic arms for their activities of daily living and independence, making their choices related to prosthesis design emphasize reliability, operational control, and prehension. As a result, BP systems are often recommended as the primary set of prostheses. Even with a functional set of prosthetic arms, additional modifications to home and work are necessary for independence. If a BP set of arms proves unable to meet basic functional needs, additional prostheses with external power, hybrid power, and/or are activity specific may be indicated.

CHOOSING TO GO WITHOUT

First and foremost, it must be acknowledged that choosing not to wear a prosthesis is perfectly acceptable as long as it is a choice. For people with upper extremity amputations, the best arm prosthesis available today still cannot feel the warmth and texture of a gentle caress. Wheelchair ambulation or crutches may be the best option when compared with the high energetic cost of ambulation with a prosthesis (or prostheses) for someone who has a high-level lower extremity amputation, bilateral amputations, or who is systemically compromised. However, before one is resigned to living one handed in a 2-handed world or going without a lower limb prosthesis, they should at least be given the opportunity to try using a prosthesis if indicated. They then have the ability to make an informed decision about when to wear, or not wear, an artificial limb.

SUMMARY

The definition of success in prosthetic rehabilitation is variable. If a person with an amputation has a prosthesis designed for weight lifting that they use for 45 minutes a day, 3 times a week and it allows them the ability to exercise, a successful outcome has been achieved. If a prosthesis is designed to allow someone to work in an industrial job for 40 hours a week but it is only tolerable for 38 hours, that is an unsuccessful outcome. Success must be defined on an individual basis.

Prosthetic rehabilitation is also nonlinear. Amputated limbs must heal. To get beyond grief, one must go through grief. Progress will be made and progress will be lost. Individuals who use a prosthesis must learn how to operate and maintain their prosthesis. As balance is recovered and residual limbs change, so too must the prosthesis be altered or replaced. Physical, occupational, and often mental health therapy are critical to facilitating the adjustment to one's disability and optimizing the remaining anatomy and physiologic reserves in preparation for prosthetic fitting and training.

Careful attention must be paid to the realistic expectations of everyone involved to prevent rejection and disappointment. Every member of the rehabilitation team is responsible for identifying and accurately setting expectations. On the day of prosthetic delivery, if patients' expectations exceed that which the clinical team can deliver, serious problems arise. If patients' expectations are set at or less than that which the clinical team can deliver, prosthetic rehabilitation will result in optimal outcomes and success.

Although this article details the numerous options that exist for individuals with amputations, the choices that determine the type of prosthesis someone wears, if they choose to wear one, must be made in consideration of specific goals and in conjunction with a rehabilitation team. The undercurrent that must be acknowledged for every person who receives a prosthesis is that the device itself is neither a magic salve that, once received and perfected, will restore them to who they were before their amputation nor a superhuman technology that will transform them into a bionic woman or man. The prosthesis is simply a component of an overall rehabilitation plan that is centered around the person with the amputation and requires a team of health care professionals in order to successfully execute.

REFERENCES

1. Board W, Street GM, Caspers C. A comparison of transtibial amputee suction and vacuum socket conditions. Prosthet Orthot Int 2001;25:202–9.
2. Goswami J, Lynn R, Street G, et al. Walking in a vacuum-assisted socket shifts the stump fluid balance. Prosthet Orthot Int 2003;27(2):107–13.
3. Gerschutz MJ, Denune JA, Colvin JM, et al. Elevated vacuum suspension influence on lower limb amputee's residual limb volume at different vacuum pressure settings. J Prosthet Orthot 2010;22(4):252–6.
4. Sanders JE, Harrison DS, Myers TR, et al. Effects of elevated vacuum on in-socket residual limb fluid volume: case study results using bioimpedance analysis. J Rehabil Res Dev 2011;48(10):1231–48.
5. Hoskins RD, Sutton EE, Kinor D, et al. Using vacuum-assisted suspension to manage residual limb wounds in persons with transtibial amputation: a case series. Prosthet Orthot Int 2013. [Epub ahead of print].
6. Pantall A, Ewins D. Muscle activity during stance phase of walking: comparison of males with transfemoral amputation with osseointegrated fixations to nondisabled male volunteers. J Rehabil Res Dev 2013;50(4):499–514.
7. Rosenbaum-Chou T. Update on osseointegration for prosthetic attachment. Academy Today 2013;9(2):A9–11.
8. American Orthotic and Prosthetic Association. AOPA prosthetic foot project report. 2010. Available at: http://www.aopanet.org/Prosthetic_Foot_Project.pdf.
9. Czerniecki JM. Research and clinical selection of foot-ankle systems. J Prosthet Orthot 2005;17(4S):35–7.
10. Daher R. Physical response of SACH feet under laboratory testing. Bull Prosthet Res 1975;10–23(Spring):4–50.
11. Sowell T. A preliminary clinical evaluation of the Mauch hydraulic foot-ankle system. Prosthet Orthot Int 1981;5(2):87–91.
12. Herr HM, Grabowski AM. Bionic ankle-foot prosthesis normalizes walking gait for persons with leg amputation. Proc Biol Sci 2012;279(1728):457–64. http://dx.doi.org/10.1098/rspb.2011.1194. PubMed PMID: 21752817; PubMed Central PMCID: PMCPMC3234569.
13. Williams RM, Turner AP, Orendurff M, et al. Does having a computerized prosthetic knee influence cognitive performance during amputee walking? Arch Phys Med Rehabil 2006;87(7):989–94. http://dx.doi.org/10.1016/j.apmr.2006.03.006. PubMed PMID: 16813788.
14. Hafner BJ, Willingham LL, Buell NC, et al. Evaluation of function, performance, and preference as transfemoral amputees transition from mechanical to microprocessor control of the prosthetic knee. Arch Phys Med Rehabil 2007;88(2):207–17. http://dx.doi.org/10.1016/j.apmr.2006.10.030. PubMed PMID: 17270519.
15. Greene MP. Four bar linkage knee analysis. Orthotics and Prosthetics 1983;37(1):15–24.
16. Saunders M, Inman V, Eberhart H. The major determinants in normal and pathological gait. J Bone Joint Surg Am 1953;35(3):543–58.

17. Gard SA, Childress DS. The influence of stance-phase knee flexion on the vertical displacement of the trunk during normal walking. Arch Phys Med Rehabil 1999; 80(1):26–32.
18. Ebrahimzadeh MH, Rajabi MT. Long-term outcomes of patients undergoing war-related amputations of the foot and ankle. J Foot Ankle Surg 2007;46(6):429–33.
19. Ephraim PL, Wegener ST, MacKenzie EJ, et al. Phantom pain, residual limb pain, and back pain in amputees: results of a national survey. Arch Phys Med Rehabil 2005;86(10):1910–9.
20. Wolf EJ, Everding VQ, Linberg AL, et al. Assessment of transfemoral amputees using C-Leg and Power Knee for ascending and descending inclines and steps. J Rehabil Res Dev 2012;49(6):831–42.
21. Wolf EJ, Everding VQ, Linberg AA, et al. Comparison of the power knee and C-Leg during step-up and sit-to-stand tasks. Gait Posture 2013;38(3):397–402. Available at: http://dx.doi.org/10.1016/j.gaitpost.2013.01.007.
22. Nelson LM, Carbone NT. Functional outcome measurements of a veteran with a hip disarticulation using a Helix 3D hip joint: a case report. J Prosthet Orthot 2011;23(1):21–6.
23. Cocchiarella L, Andersson GB, editors. Guides to the evaluation of permanent impairment. 5th edition. Chicago: AMA Press; 2001.
24. Kyberd PJ, Lemaire ED, Scheme E, et al. Two-degree-of-freedom powered prosthetic wrist. J Rehabil Res Dev 2010;48(6):609–17.
25. Lee S, Saridis G. The control of a prosthetic arm by EMG pattern recognition. IEEE Trans Automat Contr 1984;29(4):290–302.
26. Wirta RW, Taylor DR, Finley FR. Pattern recognition arm prosthesis: a historical perspective-a final report. Bull Prosthet Res 1978;10(30):8–35.
27. Scheme E, Englehart K. Electromyogram pattern recognition for control of powered upper-limb prostheses: state of the art and challenges for clinical use. J Rehabil Res Dev 2010;48(6):643–59.
28. Hargrove LJ, Lock BA, Simon AM, editors. Pattern recognition control outperforms conventional myoelectric control in upper limb patients with targeted muscle reinnervation. Engineering in Medicine and Biology Society (EMBC), 2013 35th Annual International Conference of the IEEE. Osaka, Japan, 3–7 July, 2013: IEEE.
29. Radmand A, Scheme E, Kyberd P, et al. Investigation of optimum pattern recognition methods for robust myoelectric control during dynamic limb movement. Evaluation 1500:12. May, 2013.
30. Du L, Zhang F, He H, et al, editors. Improving the performance of a neural-machine interface for prosthetic legs using adaptive pattern classifiers. Engineering in Medicine and Biology Society (EMBC), 2013 35th Annual International Conference of the IEEE. Osaka, Japan, 3–7 July, 2013: IEEE.
31. Hargrove LJ, Simon AM, Lipschutz R, et al. Non-weight-bearing neural control of a powered transfemoral prosthesis. J Neuroeng Rehabil 2013;10:62. http://dx.doi.org/10.1186/1743-0003-10-62. PubMed PMID: WOS:000321580300001.

Devising the Prosthetic Prescription and Typical Examples

Thomas Passero, AS, CP[a,b,*]

KEYWORDS

- Functional "K" levels • Terminal devices • Quality of life • Interface
- Functional aesthetic

KEY POINTS

- Limb deficiency has a significant impact on the involved person, with upper limb absence presenting a materially different set of issues than lower limb absence.
- The prescription criteria for both populations are dependent on factors beyond the anatomic involvement, or level of the deficiency.
- Although not quite reaching the definition of "controversial," there is disagreement and variability within the rehabilitation community as to the approaches taken regarding the type, timing, and combination of devices prescribed.
- In addition, there are guidelines provided by the Center for Medicare Services (CMS) and other payers that impact prescription development.

STATISTICAL SNAPSHOT

Excluding military populations, and including acquired and congenital limb absence, it is estimated that in the United States there are approximately 1.7 million people living with limb loss.[1] It is also estimated that 1 out of every 200 people in the United States has had an amputation.[2]

The main cause of acquired limb loss is poor circulation from arterial disease, with more than half occurring in patients with diabetes mellitus (**Fig. 1**). Amputation may also occur after a traumatic event or for the treatment of bone cancer. This is in contrast to congenital limb deficiency, where a person is born with complete or partial absence of a limb. It has also been documented that congenital upper limb deficiency occurs 1.6 times more often than lower limb (**Fig. 2**).[3]

Both companies are providers of upper and lower limb prostheses and related services.
[a] Prosthetic and Orthotic Program, Northwestern University Medical School, USA; [b] Handspring Upper Limb Prosthetic Specialists, Prosthetic & Orthotic Associates, Inc, Headquarters, 4 Riverside Drive, Middletown, NY 19941, USA
* Prosthetic and Orthotic Program, Northwestern University Medical School.
E-mail addresses: tom.passero@myhandspring.com; tom@poaprosthetics.com

Phys Med Rehabil Clin N Am 25 (2014) 117–132
http://dx.doi.org/10.1016/j.pmr.2013.09.009
1047-9651/14/$ – see front matter © 2014 Elsevier Inc. All rights reserved.

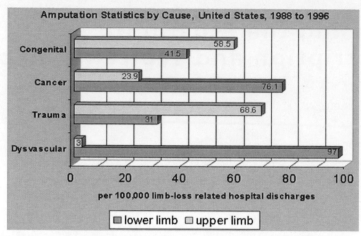

Fig. 1. Amputation statistics by cause: limb loss in the United States. (*Data from* Refs[1,2]; and Dillingham TR, Pezzin LE, MacKenzie EJ. Limb amputation and limb deficiency: epidemiology and recent trends in the United States. South Med J 2002;95:875–83.)

CONTRAINDICATIONS

For lower limb amputees, various factors can present as barriers to initiating prosthetic prescription and fitting, with some manifesting immediately postoperatively and others in the days, weeks, and months that follow. Among the postsurgical complications that present contraindications for early prosthetic consideration are the following:

- Blood loss requiring transfusion
- Deep vein thrombosis

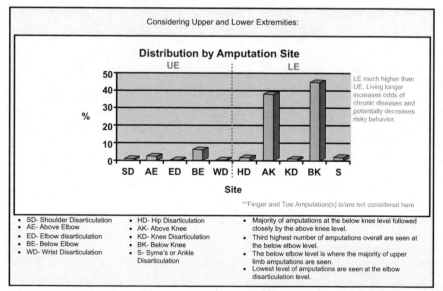

Fig. 2. Incidence per level of amputation. (*From* Highsmith MJ. Epidemiology and statistics associated with limb loss and limb deficiency. Demonstration Project on Prosthetics & Orthotics, University of South Florida College of Medicine School of Physical Therapy & Rehabilitation Sciences. Available at http://oandp.health.usf.edu/Pros/epidemiology/Final%20Epidemiology andStatistics.pdf.)

- Pulmonary embolism
- Cardiac complications including arrhythmia, congestive heart failure, and myocardial infarction
- Systemic complications including pneumonia, renal failure, stroke, and sepsis.
- Complications at the surgical site include hemorrhage or hematoma, wound infection, and failure to heal requiring additional operative interventions, such as split-thickness skin grafting, hematoma evacuation, soft tissue debridement, stump revision, and conversion to above knee amputation after below knee amputation.[4]

Among the conditions that manifest postoperatively that can become contraindications or that complicate successful prosthetic fitting are joint contractures, neuromas, severe phantom pain, reflex sympathetic dystrophy, bursitis, and tendonitis.[5] There are other skin and soft tissue complications that are potential contraindications to prosthetic prescription, but that can in many instances be overcome using creative prosthetic socket designs and/or compensating interface material. These conditions include thin and inelastic "brittle" diabetic skin, or skin and soft tissue compromised by burns, inelastic grafts, tissue adhesion, or severe scarring. Lastly, inadequate cognitive abilities or poor compliance can also obstruct successful prosthetic use.

LEVELS OF INVOLVEMENT

The level and length of the involved limb provide a basic anatomic guide to prescription development (**Fig. 3**). From superior to inferior levels for upper and lower limb involvement, the generally accepted descriptive terms are as follows:

Upper limb
a. Forequarter
b. Shoulder disarticulation
c. Transhumeral, or above elbow

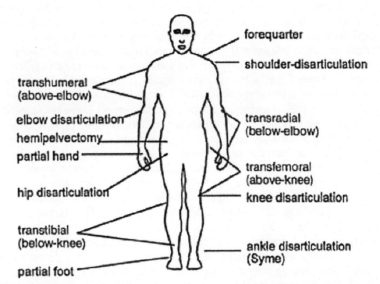

Fig. 3. A depiction of acquired amputation levels; the new ISO terms; and where applicable, the previously accepted terms. (*From* Schuch MC, Pritham CH. International Standards Organization terminology: application to prosthetics and orthotics. JPO Journal of Prosthetics & Orthotics 1994;6:31; with permission.)

    d. Elbow disarticulation
    e. Transradial or below elbow
    f. Wrist disarticulation
    g. Partial hand
    h. Digital/finger/thumb
Lower limb
    a. Hip disarticulation
    b. Transfemoral or above knee
    c. Knee disarticulation
    d. Transtibial or below knee
    e. Syme
    f. Partial foot
- Hindfoot
  - Boyd
  - Pirigoff
- Forefoot
  - Toes (typically at the metatarsophalangeal joint)
  - Transmetatarsal
  - Lisfranc
  - Chopart

CONSULTATION, MANAGING EXPECTATIONS

The benefits of a patient-centered multidisciplinary "team" management of amputee rehabilitation, including development of prescription criteria, cannot be overstated. Recent comprehensive analysis of this approach reinforces its importance in any setting, institutional or otherwise.[6]

In an institutional setting, such as a rehabilitation hospital or a rehabilitation department within a hospital, opportunities to apply these principles take place in a regularly scheduled amputee clinic, or in some form of periodic rounds. The formally assembled rehabilitation team consisting of the medical doctor and specialists in each of the allied health disciplines brings unique and mutually respected knowledge of their particular specialty to the discussion, ultimately reaching consensus on the optimal preprosthetic and prosthetic treatment plan, which is then formally "prescribed" by the physician.

In the more common private practice environment, efforts to apply these same principles should be considered as the prescription is developed. Because in most cases the team is not necessarily working in the same location, a more practical sequence of events prescribed by the managing physiatrist or surgeon is to first refer the patient to experienced clinical specialists for a prosthetic consultation or occupational and physical therapy consultation and evaluation. Using common methods of sharing of electronic medical records, and/or other communication pathways (email, Skype, GoToMeeting, and so forth), the clinical notes and other relevant information can be shared as it would in the formal rehabilitation team, providing cooperatively developed and appropriate results.

Developing an understanding of and subsequently managing the expectations of the patient and family also contribute to achieving a successful outcome. This is best accomplished with the help of an experienced prosthetist capable of discussing and demonstrating the various foot, ankle, and knee systems for the lower extremity amputee, and the components of an upper limb prosthetic system and the variety of joint and terminal devices (TDs) available for their level of involvement. In upper and lower limb cases, methods of attachment or linkage of the device to the affected limb, and realistic timelines for staged and progressive use, training, and ultimately integration of the prosthesis into their daily activities should also be covered topics.

BALANCING FUNCTION AND FORM

Comprehensive prescription development process takes into consideration the relative importance to the patient of the polarized elements of function and form. Consistent with this fact is the fundamental premise that any and all prosthetic solutions involve some level of compromise, trading elements of function for more realistic appearance, and vice versa. Identifying the patients' priorities, based on their anticipated use at home, work, and/or during recreational activities, they can more readily understand and ultimately accept these tradeoffs. Discussion of these essential compromises repeatedly by various members of the rehabilitation team early in the preprosthetic period prepares the patient and family for a successful and acceptable outcome.

No currently available technology can accomplish these polarized goals in one device. It is safe to assume that higher-functioning systems, whether for upper or lower limb, sacrifice elements of aesthetic realism for functional capability. Although the appearance of lower extremity prosthesis can be more easily hidden under clothing than an upper limb device, the shape and appearance of lower extremity prosthesis can also be important to lower limb amputees. When the appearance is not important to the wearer, the choice is often made to leave the components uncovered and therefore more visible. Ultimately these opposing factors in the equation are understood and accepted by the patient and family, and incorporated into an optimally devised prosthetic prescription.

LOWER LIMB

The transtibial and transfemoral levels of amputation make up approximately 85% of the amputee population, with the estimated proportions being 45% transtibial and 40% transfemoral.[7] As with all contemporary lower limb prostheses, the components are modular, meaning that they can be interchanged or replaced individually. The socket, knee, shin, foot, and ankle components are able to be placed and replaced independently, based on various factors. These factors can include a socket replacement for the new amputee, based on predictable volume decreases associated with muscle atrophy and reduction of postoperative edema within the first months of use, or weight changes at any time during the period of use. The knee, ankle, or foot can also be changed if and when the functional level or their weight suggests doing so. Component choices are fundamentally based on the projected or otherwise documented functional level and weight of the patient. In addition, the component choice is also influenced by the anatomic length of the affected limb, with consideration given to placing the articulation of the mechanical prosthetic joint in an optimal location relative to the normal location of the joint articulation.

Generally speaking, the longer the remnant limb, whether femur or tibia/fibula, the more limited the choice of components that fits into the space between the patient's distal limb and the knee, or the floor, without affecting joint location, leg length, stability, and balance.

UPPER LIMB

The statistical dominance of lower limb amputees over upper limb involvement is among several factors that prescribing physicians should consider when treating this population. The small numbers of upper limb involved persons relative to the numbers of clinicians treating amputees in general results in an equally small group of clinicians with adequate experience in upper limb fittings. The clinical specialties affected by this include prosthetists and occupational therapists (OTs), and physiatrists and surgeons, only a few of whom can reasonably be expected to have a depth of experience in treating them. Therefore, as part of the prescription development for upper limb amputees, it is even more important to involve prosthetists who specialize in upper limb prosthetic care and OTs with experience in evaluating and training these patients in their use. When possible, peer support provided by active users of upper limb systems can also be very useful.

It is estimated that 20% of upper limb amputees do not use their prosthetic devices,[8] with the most prevalent reason being that the device did not meet their expectations and goals. The value of prescribing an occupational therapy and prosthetic evaluation and consultation early in the case of an acquired upper limb amputation, or at any time when considering upper limb prostheses for congenitally involved upper limb absences, cannot be overstated. A prosthetist capable of demonstrating what the various types of prostheses can and cannot do helps the patient and family align their expectations with the actual functional potential of the prostheses being considered.

At this time, even the most sophisticated electronic prosthetic technology cannot reproduce the complex functions of the human hand. Referring to the prosthetic TD as tools rather than hands is useful in this regard, guiding the patient toward a realistic expectation of the functional potential of the device. Multiple tools (ie, TDs) can be prescribed, and in combination are able to perform a wide range of functional characteristics of a natural hand, including one that represents normal appearance, in shape, color, and detail, and that can also perform nongrasping functional activities.

Types of Upper Limb Prostheses

There are four general categories of upper limb prostheses: (1) body (cable) powered; (2) external (battery) powered; (3) functional aesthetic (passive); and (4) utilitarian/activity specific. A fundamental premise of contemporary upper limb prosthetic management is that no single prosthesis addresses the multiple deficits associated with upper limb loss or congenital limb deficiency. In accordance with this premise, within the equation of a prosthetic prescription should be the following factors: the level of anatomic involvement, the projected use patterns associated with the user's age, their occupation, their cognitive abilities, and avocations, all of which combine to equal functional independence. This often results in more than one prosthesis or multiple TDs being prescribed for upper limb involved persons.

Body powered

Body-powered prostheses rely on voluntary motion of a part or parts of the body, which when connected to a system of harnessing and cabling, create movement in the component parts of the system. Body-powered prostheses are simpler, weigh less, are less expensive, are more durable, and also provide some proprioceptive feedback when compared with electromechanical/myoelectic systems. Typically, they are also less aesthetic than their functional aesthetic and electronic counterparts, but are of unquestionable value as a prosthetic option. Their lack of dependence on batteries and electronics makes them more reliable and at less risk of failure when exposed to moisture or other environmental degradation.

External powered

External-powered devices consist of electromechanical articulating elements. They are able to reproduce the articulation of a single digit, pronation or supination at the wrist, and flexion and extension at the elbow. Although under development in research settings, commercially available shoulder joints are incapable at this time of powered motion (ie, flexion, extension, abduction/adduction, rotation), but are capable of powered locking and unlocking, once positioned. Finally, there are an assortment of TDs that duplicate multiple grasping patterns used for apprehending and maintaining grasp of objects of various shapes and sizes. As part of this potentiality, individual movement of single digits can be programed into the TDs for expressive and functional activities, such as pointing or using a keyboard.

Functional aesthetic (passive)

"Functional aesthetic" is a more accurate term used to describe what had formerly been described as "cosmetic" prostheses. It was not until 1998 that it was documented that "prostheses that might be considered to be worn for purely cosmetic reasons are in fact used functionally when performing everyday tasks."[9] These passive, or nonarticulating prostheses are capable of performing nongrasping activities, such as supporting, pushing, pulling, stabilizing, and balancing, and also in a supportive role when performing bimanual activities. The contradictions associated with both the definition of the word cosmetic, and the mistakenly assumed lack of function of these devices has resulted in a redefinition of this type of device.

Consideration given to the realistic appearance of prosthetic devices, in particular for the upper limb amputee, should not be considered a cosmetic element. "The concept that prostheses mimicking normal appearance are somehow nonfunctional is obsolete. Aesthetic prostheses should be provided whenever appropriate to address the intertwined functional and psychosocial deficits experienced by individuals with limb loss."[10]

Utilitarian/activity specific

In this category are the highly specific tools that can be interchangeably attached to a prosthetic system for a single activity. These include tools for the kitchen, such as knives, whisks, and pizza cutters, or for the garage, such as wrenches and files. Lastly, for recreational activities, items such as guitar picks and sports-specific adaptors for holding ski poles, baseball bats, and fishing poles to name a few can complete an array of useful items that in combination allow the user to perform vital activities that contribute to their overall quality of life.

Overuse Syndrome or Repetitive Stress Injury

"Overuse syndrome" or "repetitive stress injury" are terms that are applied to the condition that potentially affects upper limb amputees after years of one-handed activities. Symptoms of pain can manifest in all of the joints and articulations of the sound side, sometimes requiring pharmaceutical treatment and in more severe cases surgical intervention. In either case, it can impair or immobilize the upper limb involved person. Although inadequately studied or documented by clinical research, "The upper limb amputee is at risk for overuse syndrome at some point in his or her life. Although this is recognized by most prosthetists, there is currently no empiric research available to support the prevalence of overuse injuries in upper limb amputees, nor is there any research that addresses how to recognize and treat overuse symptoms before they become serious injuries in this patient population."[11]

PHYSICAL AND OCCUPATIONAL THERAPY

Typically, the physical therapist and OT spend more time with the patient than any other team members. Their roles ascend in importance as the process of preprosthetic and postprosthetic treatment unfolds. "The prosthetist and the physical therapist, as members of the rehabilitation team, often develop a very close relationship when working together with lower-limb amputees."[12] Therefore, the flow of information and patient progress among the team members radiate from the physical therapist and OT as the patient receives training, meeting the appropriate goals set in their rehabilitation plan, and eventually being discharged from care.

Much has been documented about the impact of occupational therapy in relation to prosthetic evaluation, training, and rehabilitation. In particular, for the upper limb amputee, the role of the OT has never been more important.[13]

Given the relatively recent development of more complex multiarticulating TDs, including body-powered and external-powered articulating digits for the partial hand amputee, occupational therapy has become fundamental to the achievement of successful outcomes when these devices are prescribed. The knowledge and skills required for effective OT support have migrated from responsibility for training the user in the care and maintenance of the device, independent donning and doffing, and basic use in activities of daily living, to include far more complex task training associated with the complexity of the devices being fitted.

CONGENITAL AND ACQUIRED

There are fundamental differences in the experience of persons with congenitally involved limb absence compared with those with an acquired amputation. Successful compensatory techniques are commonly developed by upper limb–deficient individuals, given that their limb deficiency is part of their lifelong normal experience. For the acquired amputee, the disability is perceived as more severe and dramatic, given their lifelong experience of two-handed engagement of objects when performing their daily tasks.

Treating the pediatric limb-deficient person, whether congenital or acquired, usually involves treating the entire family, and can ideally extend into the school and peer environment. An OT experienced in upper limb amputee treatment can contribute invaluable perspective to the patient and family through awareness of basic developmental stages, individual learning styles, social rituals, and psychosocial aspects of normal and limb-deficient persons. Knowledge and communication of these elements can and should contribute to prosthetic prescription development.

The timing of provision of prosthetic devices to congenital and acquired limb-deficient persons is also a consideration, amid some controversy. Some research indicates that there is a "Golden Period" determined to be within the first 30 days after amputation, after which the likelihood of successful adaptation to the upper limb prosthesis decreases.[14]

There are also less well documented but multiple examples of amputees having rejected prosthetic use early in their period of acquired involvement, but who in some cases decades later accept and actively use prostheses on a daily basis. The related factors that need further study are advancements in design and function, more comfortable fitting techniques, and aggressive use of OT throughout the process.

SOCKET DESIGN, LINERS, AND SUSPENSION

Similar to advances in component design described previously, design of the socket of the prosthesis has also evolved in the recent past. The patella tendon bearing socket for transtibial amputees and the quadrilateral socket design for transfemoral amputees have evolved to include such descriptions as "total surface bearing" and "ischial containment," or the most recently introduced High Fidelity[15] socket (Biodesigns Inc, Westlake Village, CA). Socket design and materials used in manufacturing are often dependent on the experience and training of the prosthetist, and his or her relative success with the various designs. Regardless of the particular design, the goals are comfort, stability, and ability to don and doff as independently as possible.

Socket liners or interfaces have multiple functions when engaging the amputee's residuum to the socket. A wide variety of silicone and nonsilicone interface materials can be used that enhance comfort by reducing shear and direct pressures to the skin and soft tissue, and provide suspension or linkage of the prosthesis to the patient's body by a mechanical locking connection. Although there are too many alternatives to outline in this article, the general categories are suction, with or without the use of a liner and locking pin; vacuum-assisted suspension systems; anatomic contour; and straps or belts.

ECONOMICS AND REIMBURSEMENT

The cost of prosthetic components has risen along with all other health care costs in the United States. Partly responsible is the application of advanced technology, such as microprocessors, hydraulics, and electromagnetic control systems. These innovations have made prostheses safer, using onboard sensors that trigger, similar to a quadriceps contraction in an intact leg, the process of stumble recovery to avoid falling. These sensors also aid the user when ascending and descending stairs and ramps, reducing the demand for oxygen and energy on what are often compromised cardiopulmonary systems. They are also stronger and lighter in weight, manufactured with such metals as aircraft aluminum and titanium, and nonmetal components composed of strong, flexible carbon fiber. Many knee and ankle components are software driven and programmable, and therefore more complicated because they more realistically reproduce the functions of the muscles and joints of the missing limbs.

Although the current reimbursement and regulatory environment related to prosthetic coverage has some fixed elements, there are also less clearly defined and more flexible guidelines still in place, unique to the contract policies of private payers. Recent passage of the Affordable Care Act presents many changes that are still uncertain in this regard. There is also a trend toward the integration of the guidelines and policies of Center for Medicare Services/Durable Medical Equipment, Prosthetics, Orthotics and Supplies into the private insurance sector, which will eventually make government and private sector guidelines more consistent.

For lower limb amputees, Center for Medicare Services/Durable Medical Equipment, Prosthetics, Orthotics and Supplies has developed a Lower Limb Prosthetic Policy, the guidelines of which tie the use of specific prosthetic components to patient functional or "K" levels defined by classifications K-0 through K-4. A basic outline of the policy, revised in March of 2013, follows:

A determination of the medical necessity for certain components/additions to the prosthesis is based on the beneficiary's potential functional abilities. Potential functional ability is based on the reasonable expectations of the prosthetist and treating physician, considering factors including, but not limited to:

1. The beneficiary's past history (including prior prosthetic use if applicable).
2. The beneficiary's current condition, including the status of the residual limb and the nature of other medical problems.
3. The beneficiary's desire to ambulate.
4. Clinical assessments of beneficiary rehabilitation potential must be based on the following classification levels:
   - Level K-0: Does not have the ability or potential to ambulate or transfer safely with or without assistance and a prosthesis does not enhance their quality of life or mobility

Patient Information

Patient Name (Last, First, MI)	Patient ID	Patient DOB	Device Type
Sample, I'm, A	0	06/03/1938	**Right Transtibial**

K Level

K2 Functional Level 2: The patient has the ability or potential for ambulation with the ability to traverse low level environmental barriers such as curbs, stairs, or uneven surfaces. Typical of the limited community ambulatory.

L-Code	Qty	Description
L5301	1	BELOW KNEE, MOLDED SOCKET, SHIN, SACH FOOT, ENDOSKELETAL SYSTEM
L5620	2	ADDITION TO LOWER EXTREMITY, TEST SOCKET, BELOW KNEE
L5637	1	ADDITION TO LOWER EXTREMITY, BELOW KNEE, TOTAL CONTACT
L5671	1	ADDITION TO LOWER EXTREMITY, BELOW KNEE / ABOVE KNEE SUSPENSION LOCKING MECHANISM (SHUTTLE, LANYARD OR EQUAL), EXCLUDES SOCKET INSERT
L5910	1	ADDITION, ENDOSKELETAL SYSTEM, BELOW KNEE, ALIGNABLE SYSTEM
L5940	1	ADDITION, ENDOSKELETAL SYSTEM, BELOW KNEE, ULTRA-LIGHT MATERIAL (TITANIUM, CARBON FIBER OR EQUAL)
L5704	1	CUSTOM SHAPED PROTECTIVE COVER, BELOW KNEE
L8470	6	PROSTHETIC SOCK, SINGLE PLY, FITTING, BELOW KNEE, EACH
L8420	6	PROSTHETIC SOCK, MULTIPLE PLY, BELOW KNEE, EACH
L5673	2	ADDITION TO LOWER EXTREMITY, BELOW KNEE/ABOVE KNEE, CUSTOM FABRICATED FROM EXISTING MOLD OR PREFABRICATED, SOCKET INSERT, SILICONE GEL, ELASTOMERIC OR EQUAL, FOR USE WITH LOCKING MECHANISM

Prescription

Projected Monthly Frequency	Estimated Length of Need
Daily	**Lifetime**
Insurance/Medicare Info	Diagnosis	Start Date **9/3/2013**
	Amputation Below Knee	ICD-9 **V49.75**
Physician Name	Physician Address	Physician UPIN
Physician Work Phone	Physician Fax	Physician NPI
( ) -	( ) -	

The above procedures and any repair and/or parts to maintain proper fit and function are appropriate for this patient, and are deemed medically necessary.

_____   Signature

_____   **Date**

_____   Print Name

Fig. 4. Orthotic and prosthetic prescription for a 75-year-old woman with diabetic-related transtibial amputation. (*Courtesy of Prosthetic & Orthotic Associates, Inc, Middletown, NY.*)

- Level K-1: Has the ability or potential to use a prosthesis for transfers or ambulation on level surfaces at fixed cadence. Typical of the limited and unlimited household ambulator.
- Level K-2: Has the ability or potential for ambulation with the ability to traverse low level environmental barriers such as curbs, stairs or uneven surfaces. Typical of the limited community ambulator.
- Level K-3: Has the ability or potential for ambulation with variable cadence. Typical of the community ambulator who has the ability to traverse most environmental barriers and may have vocational, therapeutic, or exercise activity that demands prosthetic utilization beyond simple locomotion.
- Level K-4: Has the ability or potential for prosthetic ambulation that exceeds basic ambulation skills, exhibiting high impact, stress, or energy levels. Typical of the prosthetic demands of the child, active adult, or athlete.

The records must document the beneficiary's current functional capabilities and his/her expected functional potential, including an explanation for the difference, if that is the case.

Patient Information

Patient Name (Last, First, MI)		Patient ID	Patient DOB	Device Type
Sample, I'm, A		0	09/13/1982	Right Transfemoral

K Level
K3 Functional Level 3. The patient has the ability or potential for ambulation with variable cadence. Typical of the community ambulatory who has the ability to traverse most environmental barriers and may have vocational, therapeutic, or exercise activity that demands prosthetic utilization beyond simple locomotion.

L-Code	Qty	Description
L5200	1	ABOVE KNEE, MOLDED SOCKET, SINGLE AXIS CONSTANT FRICTION KNEE, SHIN, SACH FOOT
L5624	2	ADDITION TO LOWER EXTREMITY, TEST SOCKET, ABOVE KNEE
L5631	1	ADDITION TO LOWER EXTREMITY, ABOVE KNEE OR KNEE DISARTICULATION, ACRYLIC SOCKET
L5649	1	ADDITION TO LOWER EXTREMITY, ISCHIAL CONTAINMENT/NARROW M-L SOCKET
L5650	1	ADDITIONS TO LOWER EXTREMITY, TOTAL CONTACT, ABOVE KNEE OR KNEE DISARTICULATION SOCKET
L5950	1	ADDITION, ENDOSKELETAL SYSTEM, ABOVE KNEE, ULTRA-LIGHT MATERIAL (TITANIUM, CARBON FIBER OR EQUAL)
L8430	6	PROSTHETIC SOCK, MULTIPLE PLY, ABOVE KNEE, EACH
L8480	6	PROSTHETIC SOCK, SINGLE PLY, FITTING, ABOVE KNEE, EACH
L5651	1	ADDITION TO LOWER EXTREMITY, ABOVE KNEE, FLEXIBLE INNER SOCKET, EXTERNAL FRAME
L5828	1	ADDITION, ENDOSKELETAL KNEE-SHIN SYSTEM, SINGLE AXIS, FLUID SWING AND STANCE PHASE CONTROL
L5845	1	ADDITION, ENDOSKELETAL, KNEE-SHIN SYSTEM, STANCE FLEXION FEATURE, ADJUSTABLE
L5848	1	ADDITION TO ENDOSKELETAL KNEE-SHIN SYSTEM, FLUID STANCE EXTENSION, DAMPENING FEATURE, WITH OR WITHOUT ADJUSTABILITY
L5925	1	ADDITION, ENDOSKELETAL SYSTEM, ABOVE KNEE, KNEE DISARTICULATION OR HIP DISARTICULATION, MANUAL LOCK
L5984	1	ALL ENDOSKELETAL LOWER EXTREMITY PROSTHESIS, AXIAL ROTATION UNIT, WITH OR WITHOUT ADJUSTABILITY
L5920	1	ADDITION, ENDOSKELETAL SYSTEM, ABOVE KNEE OR HIP DISARTICULATION, ALIGNABLE SYSTEM
L5673	2	ADDITION TO LOWER EXTREMITY, BELOW KNEE/ABOVE KNEE, CUSTOM FABRICATED FROM EXISTING MOLD OR PREFABRICATED, SOCKET INSERT, SILICONE GEL, ELASTOMERIC OR EQUAL, FOR USE WITH LOCKING MECHANISM
L5671	1	ADDITION TO LOWER EXTREMITY, BELOW KNEE / ABOVE KNEE SUSPENSION LOCKING MECHANISM (SHUTTLE, LANYARD OR EQUAL), EXCLUDES SOCKET INSERT
L5986	1	ALL LOWER EXTREMITY PROSTHESES, MULTI-AXIAL ROTATION UNIT (MCP' OR EQUAL)
L5987	1	ALL LOWER EXTREMITY PROSTHESIS, SHANK FOOT SYSTEM WITH VERTICAL LOADING PYLON
L5999	1	AUTOADAPTIVE MICROPROCESSOR CONTROLLED SWING & STANCE PHASE, W/ SIMULATED PHYSIOLOGICAL RULE SETS
L5999	1	DYNAMIC STABILITY CONTROL
L5999	1	LOADING FLEXED KNEE TO TRAVERSE OBSTACLES AND ASCEND STAIRS

Prescription

Projected Monthly Frequency	Estimated Length of Need	Start Date
Daily	Lifetime	2/12/2013
Insurance/Medicare Info	Diagnosis	ICD-9
	Amputation Above Knee	897.2
Physician Name	Physician Address	Physician UPIN
Physician Work Phone	Physician Fax	Physician NPI
(___) ___-____	(___) ___-____	

The above procedures and any repair and/or parts to maintain proper fit and function are appropriate for this patient, and are deemed medically necessary.

_____ Signature

_____ Date

_____ Print Name

Fig. 5. Orthotic and prosthetic prescription for a 32-year-old woman with right-side transfemoral amputation secondary to motorcycle accident. (*Courtesy of* Prosthetic & Orthotic Associates, Inc, Middletown, NY.)

It is recognized, within the functional classification hierarchy, that bilateral amputees often cannot be strictly bound by functional level classifications.[16]

The last and important fixed element of prescriptive guidelines is that all components of the prosthesis are named in the prescription.

SAMPLE PRESCRIPTIONS

What follows are four examples of software-generated prescriptions that reflect current payer guidelines and terminology. Two of them are for upper limb amputees, one transradial and one transhumeral, and two are for lower limb amputees, one transfemoral and one transtibial.

To initiate the prescriptive process, a handwritten initial prescription for "prosthetic consultation," or "above knee prosthesis" is acceptable. For the prescription that accompanies submission for payment, however, a version of what follows, which includes the CPT and alpha-numeric L-codes and the descriptive terms for each L-code component of the device, must be generated and signed.

Sample Transtibial Prescription

The prescription in **Fig. 4** is for a 75-year-old woman with diabetic-related transtibial amputation, determined to be a K-2 functional level ambulator.

A

Patient Information

| Patient Name (Last, First, MI) Sample, I'm, A | | Patient ID 0 | Patient DOB 09/13/1982 | Device Type Left Transradial |

L-Code	Qty	Description
L6935	1	BELOW ELBOW, EXTERNAL POWER, SELF-SUSPENDED INNER SOCKET, REMOVABLE FOREARM SHELL, OTTO BOCK OR EQUAL ELECTRODES, CABLES, TWO BATTERIES AND ONE CHARGER, MYOELECTRONIC CONTROL OF TERMINAL DEVICE
L7007	1	ELECTRIC HAND, SWITCH OR MYOELECTRIC CONTROLLED, ADULT
L6629	1	UPPER EXTREMITY ADDITION, QUICK DISCONNECT LAMINATION COLLAR WITH COUPLING PIECE, OTTO BOCK OR EQUAL
L6698	1	ADDITION TO UPPER EXTREMITY PROSTHESIS, BELOW ELBOW/ABOVE ELBOW, LOCK MECHANISM, EXCLUDES SOCKET INSERT
L6694	2	ADDITION TO UPPER EXTREMITY PROSTHESIS, BELOW ELBOW/ABOVE ELBOW, CUSTOM FABRICATED FROM EXISTING MOLD OR PREFABRICATED, SOCKET INSERT, SILICONE GEL, ELASTOMERIC OR EQUAL, FOR USE WITH LOCKING MECHANISM
L6687	1	UPPER EXTREMITY ADDITION, FRAME TYPE SOCKET, BELOW ELBOW OR WRIST DISARTICULATION
L6680	2	UPPER EXTREMITY ADDITION, TEST SOCKET, WRIST DISARTICULATION OR BELOW ELBOW
L7400	1	ADDITION TO UPPER EXTREMITY PROSTHESIS, BELOW ELBOW/WRIST DISARTICULATION, ULTRALIGHT MATERIAL (TITANIUM, CARBON FIBER OR EQUAL)
L7403	1	ADDITION TO UPPER EXTREMITY PROSTHESIS, BELOW ELBOW/WRIST DISARTICULATION, ACRYLIC MATERIAL
L6880	1	ELECTRIC HAND, SWITCH OR MYOELECTRIC CONTROLLED, INDEPENDENTLY ARTICULATING, DIGITS, ANY GRASP PATTERN OR COMBINATION OF GRASP PATTERNS, INCLUDES MOTOR(S)
L6890	2	ADDITION TO UPPER EXTREMITY PROSTHESIS, GLOVE FOR TERMINAL DEVICE, ANY MATERIAL, PREFABRICATED, INCLUDES FITTING AND ADJUSTMENT
L7499	1	REFERENCE L7274, PROPORTIONAL CONTROL 6-12 VOLT, UTAH OR EQUAL

Prescription

Projected Monthly Frequency Daily	Estimated Length of Need Lifetime		Start Date 9/15/2013
Insurance/Medicare Info	Diagnosis Amputation, below elbow (unilateral), without complication		ICD-9 887.0
Physician Name	Physician Address		Physician UPIN
Physician Work Phone (__) __-____	Physician Fax (__) __-____		Physician NPI

The above procedures and any repair and/or parts to maintain proper fit and function are appropriate for this patient, and are deemed medically necessary.

Signature _____   Date _____

Print Name

Fig. 6. (*A–C*) Orthotic and prosthetic prescription for a 30-year-old woman who sustained left nondominant-side traumatic amputation at mid forearm in a recreational boating accident. (*Courtesy of* Prosthetic & Orthotic Associates, Inc, Middletown, NY.)

B

Patient Information

Patient Name (Last, First, MI)		Patient ID	Patient DOB	Device Type
Sample, I'm, A		0	09/13/1982	Left Transradial

L-Code	Qty	Description
L6110	1	BELOW ELBOW, MOLDED SOCKET, (MUENSTER OR NORTHWESTERN SUSPENSION TYPES)
L6704	3	TERMINAL DEVICE, SPORT/RECREATIONAL/WORK ATTACHMENT, ANY MATERIAL, ANY SIZE
L6615	1	UPPER EXTREMITY ADDITION, DISCONNECT LOCKING WRIST UNIT
L6616	3	UPPER EXTREMITY ADDITION, ADDITIONAL DISCONNECT INSERT FOR LOCKING WRIST UNIT, EACH
L6680	2	UPPER EXTREMITY ADDITION, TEST SOCKET, WRIST DISARTICULATION OR BELOW ELBOW
L6687	1	UPPER EXTREMITY ADDITION, FRAME TYPE SOCKET, BELOW ELBOW OR WRIST DISARTICULATION
L6694	2	ADDITION TO UPPER EXTREMITY PROSTHESIS, BELOW ELBOW/ABOVE ELBOW, CUSTOM FABRICATED FROM EXISTING MOLD OR PREFABRICATED, SOCKET INSERT, SILICONE GEL, ELASTOMERIC OR EQUAL, FOR USE WITH LOCKING MECHANISM
L6698	1	ADDITION TO UPPER EXTREMITY PROSTHESIS, BELOW ELBOW/ABOVE ELBOW, LOCK MECHANISM, EXCLUDES SOCKET INSERT
L7400	1	ADDITION TO UPPER EXTREMITY PROSTHESIS, BELOW ELBOW/WRIST DISARTICULATION, ULTRALIGHT MATERIAL (TITANIUM, CARBON FIBER OR EQUAL)
L7403	1	ADDITION TO UPPER EXTREMITY PROSTHESIS, BELOW ELBOW/WRIST DISARTICULATION, ACRYLIC MATERIAL

Prescription

Projected Monthly Frequency	Estimated Length of Need		Start Date
Daily	Lifetime		9/15/2013
Insurance/Medicare Info	Diagnosis Amputation, below elbow (unilateral), without complication		ICD-9 887.0
Physician Name	Physician Address		Physician UPIN
Physician Work Phone (__) ___-____	Physician Fax (__) ___-____		Physician NPI

The above procedures and any repair and/or parts to maintain proper fit and function are appropriate for this patient, and are deemed medically necessary.

Signature _____ Date

Print Name

C

Patient Information

Patient Name (Last, First, MI)		Patient ID	Patient DOB	Device Type
Sample, I'm, A		0	09/13/1982	Left Transradial

L-Code	Qty	Description
L6400	1	BELOW ELBOW, MOLDED SOCKET, ENDOSKELETAL SYSTEM, INCLUDING SOFT PROSTHETIC TISSUE SHAPING
L6687	1	UPPER EXTREMITY ADDITION, FRAME TYPE SOCKET, BELOW ELBOW OR WRIST DISARTICULATION
L6694	2	ADDITION TO UPPER EXTREMITY PROSTHESIS, BELOW ELBOW/ABOVE ELBOW, CUSTOM FABRICATED FROM EXISTING MOLD OR PREFABRICATED, SOCKET INSERT, SILICONE GEL, ELASTOMERIC OR EQUAL, FOR USE WITH LOCKING MECHANISM
L7403	1	ADDITION TO UPPER EXTREMITY PROSTHESIS, BELOW ELBOW/WRIST DISARTICULATION, ACRYLIC MATERIAL
L7400	1	ADDITION TO UPPER EXTREMITY PROSTHESIS, BELOW ELBOW/WRIST DISARTICULATION, ULTRALIGHT MATERIAL (TITANIUM, CARBON FIBER OR EQUAL)
L6620	1	UPPER EXTREMITY ADDITION, FLEXION/EXTENSION WRIST UNIT, WITH OR WITHOUT FRICTION
L6680	2	UPPER EXTREMITY ADDITION, TEST SOCKET, WRIST DISARTICULATION OR BELOW ELBOW
L6698	1	ADDITION TO UPPER EXTREMITY PROSTHESIS, BELOW ELBOW/ABOVE ELBOW, LOCK MECHANISM, EXCLUDES SOCKET INSERT
L6703	1	TERMINAL DEVICE, PASSIVE HAND/MITT, ANY MATERIAL, ANY SIZE
L7499	1	CUSTOM HIGH DEFINITION SILICONE COVERING, LIVINGSKIN OR EQUAL

Prescription

Projected Monthly Frequency	Estimated Length of Need		Start Date
Daily	Lifetime		9/3/2013
Insurance/Medicare Info	Diagnosis Amputation, below elbow (unilateral), without complication		ICD-9 887.0
Physician Name	Physician Address		Physician UPIN
Physician Work Phone (__) ___-____	Physician Fax (__) ___-____		Physician NPI

The above procedures and any repair and/or parts to maintain proper fit and function are appropriate for this patient, and are deemed medically necessary.

Signature _____ Date

Print Name

Fig. 6. (continued)

Patient Information			
Patient Name (Last, First, MI) **Sample, I'm, A**	Patient ID 0	Patient DOB 09/13/1982	Device Type **Left Transhumeral**

L-Code	Qty	Description
L6250	1	ABOVE ELBOW, MOLDED DOUBLE WALL SOCKET, INTERNAL LOCKING ELBOW, FOREARM
L6615	1	UPPER EXTREMITY ADDITION, DISCONNECT LOCKING WRIST UNIT
L6665	1	UPPER EXTREMITY ADDITION, TEFLON, OR EQUAL, CABLE LINING
L6670	1	UPPER EXTREMITY ADDITION, HOOK TO HAND, CABLE ADAPTER
L6676	1	UPPER EXTREMITY ADDITION, HARNESS, (E.G. FIGURE OF EIGHT TYPE), DUAL CABLE DESIGN
L6682	2	UPPER EXTREMITY ADDITION, TEST SOCKET, ELBOW DISARTICULATION OR ABOVE ELBOW
L6688	1	UPPER EXTREMITY ADDITION, FRAME TYPE SOCKET, ABOVE ELBOW OR ELBOW DISARTICULATION
L6698	1	ADDITION TO UPPER EXTREMITY PROSTHESIS, BELOW ELBOW/ABOVE ELBOW, LOCK MECHANISM, EXCLUDES SOCKET INSERT
L7401	1	ADDITION TO UPPER EXTREMITY PROSTHESIS, ABOVE ELBOW DISARTICULATION, ULTRALIGHT MATERIAL (TITANIUM, CARBON FIBER OR EQUAL)
L7404	1	ADDITION TO UPPER EXTREMITY PROSTHESIS, ABOVE ELBOW DISARTICULATION, ACRYLIC MATERIAL
L6694	2	ADDITION TO UPPER EXTREMITY PROSTHESIS, BELOW ELBOW/ABOVE ELBOW, CUSTOM FABRICATED FROM EXISTING MOLD OR PREFABRICATED, SOCKET INSERT, SILICONE GEL, ELASTOMERIC OR EQUAL, FOR USE WITH LOCKING MECHANISM
L6605	1	UPPER EXTREMITY ADDITIONS, SINGLE PIVOT HINGE, PAIR
L6616	2	UPPER EXTREMITY ADDITION, ADDITIONAL DISCONNECT INSERT FOR LOCKING WRIST UNIT, EACH
L6709	1	TERMINAL DEVICE, HAND, MECHANICAL, VOLUNTARY CLOSING, ANY MATERIAL, ANY SIZE
L6722	1	TERMINAL DEVICE, HOOK OR HAND, HEAVY DUTY, MECHANICAL, VOLUNTARY CLOSING, ANY MATERIAL, ANY SIZE, LINED OR UNLINED
L6890	2	ADDITION TO UPPER EXTREMITY PROSTHESIS, GLOVE FOR TERMINAL DEVICE, ANY MATERIAL, PREFABRICATED, INCLUDES FITTING AND ADJUSTMENT

Prescription		
Projected Monthly Frequency **Daily**	Estimated Length of Need **Lifetime**	Start Date **3/15/2013**
Insurance/Medicare Info	Diagnosis **Amputation, Unilateral, Below knee, w/o complication, Amputation at or above elbow**	ICD-9 **897.0, 887.2**
Physician Name	Physician Address	Physician UPIN
Physician Work Phone ( ) -	Physician Fax ( ) -	Physician NPI

The above procedures and any repair and/or parts to maintain proper fit and function are appropriate for this patient, and are deemed medically necessary.

Signature _____

Print Name _____

Date _____

Fig. 7. Orthotic and prosthetic prescription for a 29-year-old man with dominant-side emergency department amputation from a motor vehicle accident. (*Courtesy of* Prosthetic & Orthotic Associates, Inc, Middletown, NY.)

Sample Transfemoral Prescription

The prescription in **Fig. 5** is for a 32-year-old woman with right-side transfemoral amputation secondary to a motorcycle accident. The patient is otherwise healthy and previously highly active, and was determined to be a K-3 functional level ambulator.

Sample Transradial Prescription

The prescription in **Fig. 6** is for a 30-year-old woman who sustained left nondominant side traumatic amputation at mid forearm in a recreational boating accident. A professional finance executive also active in sports and recreational activities, her three prescription were for (1) a high-definition functional aesthetic prosthesis; (2) an external-powered prosthesis with multiarticulating TD; and (3) an activity-specific prosthesis with attachments for skiing, cycling, and golfing. Three separate prescriptions were required.

Sample Transhumeral Prescription

The prescription in **Fig. 7** is for a 29-year-old man with dominant-side emergency department amputation from a motor vehicle accident. Based on history of manual work experience in a warehouse, a body-powered system was prescribed, with multiple TDs.

REFERENCES

1. Ziegler-Graham K, MacKenzie EJ, Ephraim PL, et al. Estimating the prevalence of limb loss in the United States: 2005 to 2050. Arch Phys Med Rehabil 2008;89: 422–9.
2. Adams PF, Hendershot GE, Marano MA, et al. Current estimates from the National Health Interview Survey, 1996. Vital Health Stat 10 1999;(200):1–203.
3. McGinsey G, Bradford TC. White paper from the Bioengineering Institute Center for Neuroprosthetics Worcester Polytechnic Institution 2011.
4. Standard of Care. Lower Extremity Amputation Copyright ©2011 The Brigham and Women's Hospital, Inc., Department of rehabilitation Services.
5. Knetsche RP, Leopold SS, Brage ME. Inpatient management of lower extremity amputations. Foot Ankle Clin 2001;6(2):229–41.
6. Lusardi MM, Neilsen N, Milagros JM. Orthotics and prosthetics in rehabilitation. 3rd edition. Elsevier; 2012. p. 1–13.
7. University of South Florida College of Medicine: School of Physical Therapy and Rehabilitation Sciences College of Engineering: Mechanical Engineering Department. Highsmith, Quillen and Dubey; Funded by Department of Education Rehab Services Administration, Award # H235J050020.
8. Biddiss EA, Chau TT. Upper limb prosthesis use and abandonment: a survey of the last 25 years. Prosthet Orthot Int 2007;31(3):236–57.
9. Fraser CM. An evaluation of the use made of cosmetic and functional prostheses by unilateral upper limb amputees. Prosthet Orthot Int 1998;22:216–23.
10. Doolan K, Passero T. Aesthetic prostheses. In: Smith DG, Michael JW, Bowker JH, editors. Atlas of Amputations and Limb Deficiencies. 3rd edition. Elsevier; 2004. p. 303–10.
11. Gambrell CR. Overuse syndrome and the unilateral upper limb amputee: consequences and prevention. J Prosthet Orthot 2008;20(3):126–32. http://dx.doi.org/10.1097/JPO.0b013e31817ecb16.

12. Gailey RS Jr, Clark CR. Atlas of limb prosthetics: surgical, prosthetic, and reha-bilitation principles. Physical therapy management of adult lower-limb amputees. In: Smith DG, Michael JW, Bowker JH, editors. Atlas of Amputations and Limb Deficiencies. 3rd edition. Elsevier; 2004.

13. Smurr LM, Gulick K, Yancosek K, et al. Managing the upper extremity amputee: a protocol for success. J Hand Ther 2008;21(2):160–76 Treating The War Casualty.

14. Malone JM, Fleming LL, Robertson J, et al. Immediate, early, and late postsur-gical management of upper limb amputations. J Rehabil Res Dev 1984;21:33–41.

15. Alley RD, Williams TW III, Albuquerque MJ, et al. Prosthetic sockets stabilized by alternating areas of tissue compression and release. J Rehabil Res Dev 2011; 48(6):679–96.

16. Local Coverage Determination (LCD): Lower Limb Prostheses (L11464) NHIC, Corp. LCD ID L11464 Lower Limb Prostheses Contract Number 16003; Contract Type DME MAC.

Prosthetic Training: Upper Limb

Shawn Swanson Johnson, BS, OTR/L[a],*, Elizabeth Mansfield, BA[b]

KEYWORDS

- Occupational therapy • Prosthetic training • Rehabilitation • Upper limb
- Prosthetics

KEY POINTS

- A collaborative approach is essential to successful rehabilitation.
- The choice of componentry determines the training needs.
- Prosthetic component manufacturers are a useful resource.
- Managing expectations during therapy is crucial in helping minimize client frustration.
- Mastering skills before proceeding to the next set of skills during training is vital for improved client outcomes.

INTRODUCTION

For the individual who receives an arm prosthesis, occupational therapy is a critical piece of the overall rehabilitation puzzle. An occupational therapist (OT) will help the individual learn to use their prosthesis; use it for activities of daily living (ADL); and, it is hoped, incorporate it into their everyday life. But an OT can only do so much.

If the prosthesis does not fit, is poorly designed, has components that are inappropriate, has components that are assembled incorrectly, and/or is improperly programed, then the OT will struggle greatly or will be unable to train the individual how to use their prosthesis properly. This scenario could lead to frustration for the OT and especially the individual with limb loss. Without proper knowledge of what components are appropriate or how a prosthesis is supposed to fit, individuals might think it is their fault and that they need to try harder and practice more, when ultimately this will lead nowhere. The OT, in turn, may wonder what they are doing wrong. It is imperative that there is constant collaboration and frequent communication between the certified prosthetist (CP) and the OT for the best overall outcome for individuals with an arm prosthesis.

[a] Occupational Therapy, 16111 Park Center Way, Houston, TX 77059, USA; [b] Clinical Education Concepts, 221 Fox Hill Drive, Baiting Hollow, NY 11933, USA
* Corresponding author.
E-mail address: Shawn.Swanson.Johnson@gmail.com

Phys Med Rehabil Clin N Am 25 (2014) 133–151
http://dx.doi.org/10.1016/j.pmr.2013.09.012
1047-9651/14/$ – see front matter © 2014 Elsevier Inc. All rights reserved.
pmr.theclinics.com

For the purposes of this text, this article solely focuses on adult upper limb prosthetic training. Pediatric prosthetic training will vary significantly secondary to the nature of the limb loss/limb difference. Parental involvement is a crucial factor, and training typically happens in phases according to the various developmental milestones and stages of life. Many resources are available for pediatric prosthetic training.[1–4]

TYPES OF PROSTHESES: AN OT'S PERSPECTIVE

The OT essentially needs to know that there are 5 types of prostheses and the various terms that might be used to describe the same type of prosthesis:

1. Cosmetic or passive functional
2. Body powered or cable driven
3. Electrically powered (myoelectric or switch controlled)
4. Hybrid (combination of body powered and electric)
5. Activity specific (designed for a specific task, such as swimming or showering)

But an OT should be able to rely on the CP for more detailed information regarding the various types of prostheses available for individuals with upper limb loss. Please see the article by Kistenberg elsewhere in this issue.

To properly train an individual with an arm prosthesis, the OT must understand the following:

- What type of prosthesis their patient has
- What componentry is on the prosthesis
- If electric, how the components are programed

The OT and CP should communicate on an ongoing and regular basis to discuss any questions regarding the prosthesis as well as any problems, issues, or barriers that might impede training.

WORKING CLOSELY WITH THE CP AND PROSTHETIC COMPONENT MANUFACTURER

The OT should form a close working relationship with the CP and even attend prosthetic appointments with their client if possible and when necessary. The same should go for the CP attending OT appointments because this will only help both professionals understand what it is the other is looking for and more closely appreciate each other's roles and responsibilities because some items may overlap or one professional might have a resource that the other was unaware of.

The CP has typically formed a relationship with the prosthetic component manufacturer, which is crucial with today's evolving and rapidly advancing technology. The prosthetic manufacturers offer instructional courses and training on their specific components and technology and, in some instances, require the CP to bring and fit a client in order to become a certified provider of that particular technology. The prosthetic manufacturers encourage the CPs to bring OTs to courses because this helps foster the relationship and enhances the OT's knowledge base. The OT is not required to understand all of the intricate details of the components, technology, and programing; however, the more knowledge acquired, the better they are able to train individuals how to use their prosthesis and use it in their ADL.

GOALS AND TIME FRAMES

The time from an individual being casted for a prosthesis to incorporating it into their daily life varies greatly. General time frames for prosthetic training rehabilitation are available[5]; but it is important to keep in mind that the rehabilitation time frames are dependent on many factors, which can heavily influence the time spent in therapy. Some of those factors include the following:

- Nature of limb loss/limb difference (acquired vs congenital)
- Concomitant injuries
- Level of limb loss
- Number of limbs affected
- Type of prosthesis
- Componentry used
- Programing
- Previous prosthetic wear/use
- Previous therapy
- Experience level of prosthetist
- Motivation of client
- Client cognition
- Experience level of therapist
- Availability of client
- Availability of prosthetist
- Insurance

In some cases, individuals may receive a preparatory prosthesis[6] within a day or two (typically referred to as an expedited fitting); in other cases, it may be months before they receive a definitive or finalized prosthesis. Whether an individual receives a preparatory or definitive prosthesis is up to the prosthetist. It is recommended that the OT be involved from the initial stages of the prosthetic fabrication process and begin training with a preparatory prosthesis. The OT will be able to put the client in various therapy situations, which will help determine if any modifications need to be made before the CP finalizes the prosthesis. It is easier to modify a preparatory prosthesis than a definitive prosthesis. Once training has begun, it could take anywhere from a few days to several months in order for the client to feel proficient with their prosthesis. Again, the time frame depends on the factors mentioned earlier. Managing expectations is important. The proliferation of feel-good stories in the media and online can cause/create a significant disconnect between a client's expectations and realistic expectations. Early prosthetic training is feasible if there are no outstanding preprosthetic rehabilitation areas to be addressed.

The goals of upper limb prosthetic training should be client centered and meaningful. The OT and family members may also have certain goals in mind for the client that will help them be more independent with basic self-care tasks; but if it is not meaningful to the client, then it may not be appropriate to address it in therapy because it could lead to frustration and a battle of wills. That does not mean the client will not find those tasks meaningful or important in the future, therapy tends to be a process that occurs in phases, and those tasks can always be addressed at a later time. All that being said, it is important to discuss with the client the need for independence with self-care activities in the event someone is not around to help. Some common goals the OT should keep in mind include the following:

- Independence with don/doff of the prosthesis
- Perform basic self-care tasks independently with the prosthesis or adaptive equipment (feeding, bathing, toileting, dressing)

- Perform ADL independently with the prosthesis or adaptive equipment (feeding, meal preparation, grooming, home management)
- Engage in leisure activities/hobbies with the prosthesis or adaptive equipment

OCCUPATIONAL THERAPY INITIAL ASSESSMENT

It would be ideal if the same OT performed both the preprosthetic evaluation and prosthetic training evaluation, but this may not always be the case. The preprosthetic phase of rehabilitation should have prepared the client and his or her body/limb to wear, tolerate, and use a prosthesis, which will ultimately make the prosthetic training phase much smoother and faster.

If an individual has not received any preprosthetic rehabilitation, it may make the prosthetic training phase difficult for the following reasons:

- Range of Motion (ROM) deficits
- Strength deficits
- Scar tissue adhesions
- Edema
- Hypersensitivity
- Pain issues

For example, adherent scar tissue will affect the individual's ability to wear a socket without skin breakdown. Edema or volume fluctuation in the residual limb will affect the fit of the socket and ultimately the client's comfort and/or control ROM or strength deficits will affect the individual's ability to control the various components on their prosthesis. These areas must be addressed before prosthetic training can begin, and changes to the prosthesis may be necessary once these areas have been resolved. This will be a source of frustration for both the OT and especially the client who was expecting to learn how to use their new prosthesis and instead may feel like they took 3 steps back. Please see the article by Klarich and Brueckner elsewhere in this issue.

In any event, the OT initial assessment should paint a very thorough picture of the individual and describe in detail any problem areas in order to justify what needs to be addressed during the prosthetic training phase and identify barriers to training. The areas to be addressed during the assessment should include, but are not limited to the following:

- Cause and onset
- Age, hand dominance
- Other medical issues
- Surgeries
- Medications
- Level of independence with ADL
- ROM
- Strength
- Skin integrity
- Shape of residual limb
- Phantom pain
- General pain
- School and/or work/vocational goals
- Support
- Home environment
- Previous therapies

- Previous prostheses
- Client goals

PROSTHETIC DELIVERY OVERVIEW: AN OT'S PERSPECTIVE

The OT is typically the health care professional that spends the most time with individuals with upper limb loss. Although the CP will give an overview of the componentry, explain the various features, provide education regarding prosthetic wear and care, and demonstrate how to put the prosthesis on and take it off, this might only happen when the client first receives their prosthesis. The OT should be familiar with all of the items discussed during prosthetic delivery so it can be reviewed as necessary during prosthetic training. The OT should review the following areas:

- Prosthesis wear schedule
- Skin checks
- How to take care of and clean their prosthetic socket
- Harness and components
- What hazards to avoid
- What the various components are
- How the components work/operate on their prosthesis
  - Terminal device (TD)
  - Wrist
  - Harness
  - Cables
  - Liner
  - Socket

If the prosthesis is electric, the OT should thoroughly review the various components (TD, wrist, and elbow) and how they are programmed. Once the prosthetic training begins, repetition of this information will help it sink in and make more sense.

The OT should also teach clients how to put their prosthesis, including socks and liners, on and remove it independently. There are various methods for don/doff of arm prostheses. The methods will differ depending on the type of socket, type of prosthesis, personal preference, and the level of limb loss. For someone with a body-powered prosthesis, the methods are similar to putting on or taking off a sweater or a coat. If the individual is wearing a myoelectric prosthesis, they may have a suction socket and require a pull sock to don their arm for an appropriate fit and electrode contact. If an individual is missing more than one limb, adaptive equipment may be necessary. The adaptive equipment can range from a simple work hook mounted to a wall or to a complex dressing tree for individuals with higher-level bilateral limb loss (**Figs. 1** and **2**).

WHAT TO LOOK FOR BEFORE TRAINING BEGINS

If an individual has an electrically powered prosthesis, it is important for the OT to take a few steps back and assess things at a very basic level. This assessment will help the OT determine if there are any problem areas that could impede training and lead to frustration during the actual training. Problem areas can include but are not limited to the following:

- Muscle strength and endurance
- Socket fit
- Electrode placement

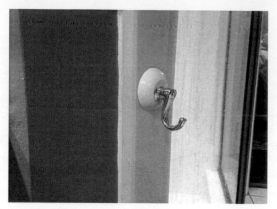

Fig. 1. Work Hook with Suction Cup. (*Courtesy of* Shawn Swanson Johnson. Skills for Life 4: Bilateral Upper Limb Loss Workshop.)

- Electrode gain settings
- Incorrect wiring
- Device programing
- Patients' general understanding/comprehension

Because of the advances in prosthetic technology hardware and software over the past 10 to 15 years, it is now possible to virtually assess an individual's ability to operate a prosthesis (**Fig. 3**).

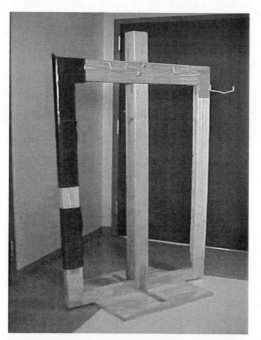

Fig. 2. Dressing tree. (*Courtesy of* Suzanne Krenek Andrews, TIRR Memorial Hermann.)

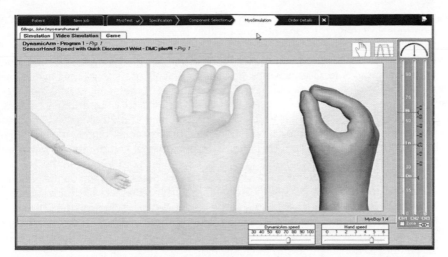

Fig. 3. Assessment of prosthesis operation. (*Courtesy of* Ottobock, Minneapolis, MN.)

VIRTUAL EVALUATION AND TRAINING

Before this technology was available, training someone with an electric prosthesis was an inexact science. Clients would put their prosthesis on; try to operate whatever componentry they had (hand, wrist, or elbow); and, if they demonstrated control, then it was time to move onto a few drills and ADL. If they did not demonstrate control, OTs, CPs, and their clients would be left to guess what the possible problems might be. Most of the time, it was assumed that the clients just needed more practice/ training. However, if the underlying problem was socket fit, electrode placement, or electrode gain settings, no amount of practice was going to help clients learn how to use their prosthesis. The ability to observe an individual's muscle strength and their ability to control a virtual prosthesis before ever being fit with an actual prosthesis now eliminates most of the guesswork. The OT will need to use a combination of computerized software and hardware that various prosthetic manufacturers offer as well as 2 electrodes with cables. The electrodes should be placed on the bulk of the muscle belly as a starting point and then moved from there to determine the most optimal muscle sites for control. The electrode gain settings should ideally start at a lower level (for example, when using an Otto Bock electrode (Duderstadt, Germany), start at a level between 2–4) because this gives an unadjusted or real view of an individual's muscle strength without any artificial strengthening of the muscles. The optimal muscle sites will depend on the following:

- Strength
- Controllability
- Endurance

In addition, the muscle sites need to fall within the trimlines of the future socket. There is no point evaluating or training muscles that fall outside of the socket area because it will only lead to frustration. Once the electrodes are determined to be properly located, adjustments to electrode gains can be made for easier and optimal control. The electrode gain should not be too high because it will be too sensitive and clients will lack the ability to control slow speeds or could inadvertently operate their wrist. The ability to control slow speeds is necessary to avoid crushing or dropping objects. The electrode gain should not be too low or clients will be unable to generate enough muscle strength to operate any of their prosthetic components. The OT is looking for clients to have natural and easy control. Clients should neither have to struggle or shake to elicit a good muscle contraction nor hold a muscle contraction for a long period of time. Clients with a higher level of limb loss should not have extraneous or exaggerated movements and should be able to isometrically isolate the muscle they want to contract. In order for clients to understand what an easy, natural contraction should feel or look like, the OT can demonstrate on themselves first and then place the electrodes on the clients' sound limb before proceeding to their residual limb. The OT should advise clients to perform the movements and/or training with both arms during the virtual assessment (**Fig. 4**). For example, in order to open the TD, clients with a transradial amputation should extend their wrist and fingers on their sound arm and also imagine doing it with their phantom wrist and fingers at the same time.

Once the muscle sites are selected and the electrodes are adjusted, the OT needs to understand how the clients' prosthetic arm is programmed. There are many different variations of programs to choose from and depending on how the client presents. Factors to consider include the following:

- Muscle strength
- Number of muscles are available for control
- Cognitive ability
- Problem-solving ability
- Level of limb loss

After the CP determines the programing and the OT understands the programing, virtual training can begin. Depending on the virtual software/hardware being used, virtual training can happen in various ways; this type of training will help strengthen the muscles sites, work on endurance, teach clients how to switch between components, and generally build confidence. It typically includes an assessment screen, fun games, and virtual prosthetic component training. On the evaluation screen, the OT can verbally cue for what they want the clients to do (for example, "Try to reach this line quickly with your wrist extensors, which is the red signal, or try to slowly contract your bicep muscle, which is the blue color, and stay under this line."). The games (car maze, manipulating balls) can be a fun way for clients to train and practice without

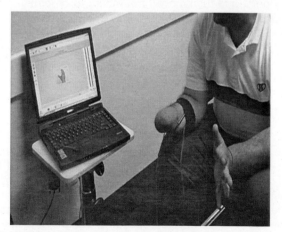

Fig. 4. Virtual training of amputee.

realizing that they are actually working. The virtual prosthetic component screen allows clients to control the various components on a computer screen, which simulates wearing a prosthesis (minus the weight). During this time, clients will learn the various nuances of how their prosthetic arm may be programed or controlled. Clients should also be advised that they do not have to hold a contraction in order to keep the TD open or closed.

Virtual training should be done sitting, standing, and in various planes of the body to demonstrate real-world scenarios; but the electrode cables can make this difficult during the evaluation phase.

If clients are successful with the virtual training, theoretically they should experience success with their actual prosthesis. This virtual training should help reduce the actual prosthetic training treatment time because the clients are already familiar with controlling a virtual prosthesis. The only major differences at this point are the fit and weight of the socket and the ability to do drills and activities while moving about the room. If clients experience problems once they have their prosthesis on, then it is time to reassess and discuss the following with the prosthetist in a collaborative manner:

- Electrode placement
- Socket fit
- Harnessing
- Componentry programing

If the electrode is not in the optimal location, it may cause problems with the controllability of the various electric components. Moving the electrode slightly (either from side to side, down/up, or adjusting the angle) may help clients elicit a stronger or more consistent signal. If the socket is not fitting comfortably and intimately, then the clients' skin may not be making appropriate contact with the electrodes in the socket. Clients will not be able to control their prosthesis consistently or accurately if the socket does not fit. The various devices may move, but it may be because the clients' skin is rubbing along the electrode causing a stray or inadvertent signal not an intentional signal meant to control a device. If clients have to sit or hold their prosthesis on with their other arm, that is a sign of an improper fit. Clear test sockets are extremely helpful during early training to problem solve.

TRAINING DEPENDS ON TYPE OF PROSTHESIS

The stages of prosthetic training are typically the same regardless of the type of prosthesis, but the nature and length of the training will differ depending on the following factors:

- Level of limb loss
- Number of limbs affected
- Type of prosthesis
- Type of components
- If electric, componentry programing

That being said, all types of prosthesis require training and, as mentioned previously, will vary based on the type of prosthesis that clients have been prescribed. For clients with a cosmetic/passive functional prosthesis, training will be minimal and include ways for individuals to stabilize or support objects. The OT will typically have clients stabilize their cosmetic arm on top of a piece of paper for writing or have clients use the cosmetic arm to support a tray of food at a restaurant. For the activity-specific prosthesis or activity-specific TD, training will also be minimal because it is particular to the activity clients want to perform, such as showering, swimming, fishing, weight training, field sports, rock climbing, and so forth. Keep in mind that activity-specific training will most likely be happening at the conclusion of their primary prosthesis training whether it is body powered, electric, or hybrid.

THREE STAGES OF UPPER LIMB PROSTHETIC TRAINING

For the body-powered, electrically powered, or the hybrid types of prosthesis, there are 3 stages of prosthetic training:

- Controls training
- Repetitive drills
- Bimanual functional skill training

These 3 stages are important building blocks for successful prosthetic training. It is not advised to have clients put on a prosthesis and have them attempt to feed or dress themselves on the first visit. This practice will lead to frustration and may cause clients to abandon their prosthesis before proper training has even begun. Clients should master each stage (95%–100% accuracy and consistency) before moving on to the next stage. This progression of training allows the therapist the ability to tease out any problem areas whether it is with the prosthesis and its components, socket or harness fit, or with the patients' physical and/or cognitive ability. If clients are having difficulty with basic operation of their components, then they are certainly going to have difficulty with grasping and releasing objects and performing 2-handed activities. The components should not be moving on their own or operating randomly and intermittently. If there is a problem in any one of the 3 stages, then the therapist can report back to the prosthetist to determine if any modifications or adjustments need to be made before moving on to the next stage. There is a method to the madness, and explaining each of the stages to clients and what to expect during each stage and why they are being done facilitates buy-in and an overall understanding of the process (**Table 1**).

Keep in mind that people complete tasks differently. How an activity is completed will depend on the patients' level of amputation and prosthetic device. Therapists typically learn more from patients than the patients learn from the therapists. The more exposure and experience a therapist has with individuals with limb loss, the more knowledge they will have to pass on to the next person. In addition, the Internet has an abundance of videos with instructional tutorials on how to complete certain tasks. Lastly, it is advisable to introduce current patients to former patients, especially if there is someone who has a similar level of limb loss and prosthetic componentry. It is invaluable for them to be able to talk to someone else who has gone through similar experiences. This communication allows the current patient to see what challenges may lie ahead, how others cope, how others complete certain activities, and so forth.

ELECTRICALLY POWERED COMPONENT SELECTION AND PROGRAMING: HOW IT AFFECTS TRAINING

Electric prosthesis training will differ slightly depending on what type of components are being used and how they are programmed. Many of the prosthetic manufacturers provide training guidelines or informational brochures with their devices or components. These guidelines are extremely helpful in better understanding the technology so the OT can explain to the clients exactly how their componentry works (see **Table 2** for manufacturer information). Also, if possible, the OT should connect themselves to

Table 1
Three stages of prosthetic training

Stage	What Does it Entail?	Purpose and How to Perform	When is it Appropriate and How Long Does it Last?
1. Controls training	• Open and close the terminal device • Rotate and/or flex and extend the wrist • Flex and extend the elbow • Position the shoulder • Control speeds • Switch between components	Simon says or mirror image of the therapist Teach the clients how to operate all of the various components on their prosthesis before introducing objects to grasp and release Look for clients to achieve consistent and accurate control; prosthesis should do what clients want it to do every time	Initial stage of prosthetic training; can last a few minutes to a few days; should be mastered before moving on to the next stage
2. Repetitive drills	• Foam or wooden therapy peg board • Stacking cones • Clothespin relocation task • Transferring blocks and balls into a bucket • Ring tree • Styrofoam or plastic cup • String beads	Should be done in sitting, standing, and walking; transferring play objects of various sizes and densities to locations of various heights and levels; practice graded grasp and release without dropping or crushing; repeat, repeat, repeat Give clients confidence the prosthesis will do what it is supposed to do in a therapy or practice situation before moving on to a 2-handed task	Initial and middle stages of prosthetic training; can last from a few hours to a few days; should be mastered before moving on to the next stage
3. Bimanual functional skill training	• Twist on/off lids • Pour water into a cup (prosthesis holding cup) • Place a pillow in a pillow case • Pack a suitcase • Wrap a present • Carry a tray • Manage money • Prepare and eat a meal • Many other meaningful bimanual ADL	Engage in tasks clients will encounter on a routine basis; should be meaningful and progress from simple to complex activities Teach clients independence in ADL using their prosthesis; forcing 2-handed situations to minimize stress on unaffected arm	Middle and end stages of prosthetic training; can last a few days to a few weeks; home and work activities should be addressed; may be done in incremental stages as new needs may arise over the course of the clients' prosthetic use

Table 2
Upper limb loss rehabilitation resources

Conferences	Videos	Upper Limb Prosthetic Manufacturers*	Continuing Education Courses	Outcome Measure Information
ISPO World Congress http://www.ispoint.org/events/world-congress	Training the Client with an Electrically Powered Prosthesis Info@UtahArm.com or (888) 696-2767	Fillauer Companies, Inc http://www.fillauercompanies.com/ Hosmer Dorrance Corporation http://hosmer.com/ Motion Control http://www.utaharm.com/	Otto Bock Academy (online tutorials, live classes, interactive webinars) http://academy.ottobockus.com/	Southampton Hand Assessment Procedure
MEC Symposium http://www.unb.ca/conferences/mec/	Skills for Life 2: Bilateral Upper Limb Loss Workshop Proceedings www.resrec.com	Liberating Technologies http://www.liberatingtech.com/	AOTA Approved Provider Program (remote and live courses) http://www.aota.org/en/Education-Careers/Continuing-Education/ForProviders.aspx	Assessment of Capacity for Myoelectric Control
Skills for Life http://www.usispo.org/skills_for_life.asp	RIC Resource Library http://lifecenter.ric.org/ Search Health care topic: medical information & care Subtopic: amputee	Otto Bock http://www.ottobockus.com	US-ISPO www.usispo.org and International ISPO http://www.ispoint.org/ispo-elearning	Box & Blocks
AAOP http://www.oandp.org/	Art Heinze Bilateral Upper Limb Loss www.armamputee.com	RSL/Steeper http://www.rslsteeper.com/	AAOP (interactive webinars, online tutorials, conferences) http://www.oandp.org/olc/	Activities Measure for Upper-Limb Amputees

AOPA www.aopanet.org/	Eric Nelson: Bilateral Upper Limb Loss ednelson@fgn.net	Texas Assistive Devices www.n-abler.org	Clinical Education Concepts (live courses) http://www.cecpo.com/	Jebsen Taylor Test of Hand Function
AOTA www.aota.org	YouTube Search Keywords: Arm amputation, Arm prosthesis, Upper limb loss rehabilitation, Upper limb loss, Upper limb prosthesis, Upper extremity prosthesis, Bilateral upper limb loss rehabilitation, Arm prosthetic device	Touch Bionics http://www.touchbionics.com/	Various prosthetic care facilities provide in-services or continuing education events Find local providers at http://www.abcop.org	Official Findings of the State of the Science Conference #9: Upper Limb Prosthetic Outcome Measures (AAOP Publication) http://www.oandp.org/jpo/library/index/2009_04S.asp
Amputee Coalition http://www.amputee-coalition.org	—	TRS, Inc http://www.oandp.com/products/trs/about/	—	Clothespin Relocation Test
—	—	Vincent Prosthetic Systems http://vincentsystems.de/en/	—	—
—	—	*This list does not include prosthetic patient care facilities that may make or be developing their own devices or products that are not commercially available	—	—

Abbreviations: AAOP, American Academy of Orthotists & Prosthetists; AOPA, American Orthotic & Prosthetic Association; AOTA, American Occupational Therapy Association; ISPO, International Society for Prosthetics and Orthotics; RIC, Rehabilitation Institute of Chicago.

the electrodes, computer software, and prosthetic hardware so they can feel what it is like and what is involved when operating a prosthetic device. Some components (hands, wrists, elbows) can be controlled proportionally, which means clients have the ability to vary the speed and/or the pinch force based on how hard or soft they contract their muscle. Other components can only be controlled with one speed despite the strength of their muscle contraction, which is often referred to as *digital control*. Some prosthetic systems have the ability to perform simultaneous control of 2 or more components (for instance, simultaneous movement of the elbow and the terminal device), whereas others require clients to switch between components by eliciting a certain muscle signal or using an external physical switch. There are several options to choose from when switching between components, and they can be tested out virtually or during prosthetic training to see which modes clients perform better with. Two of the most common modes of switching are typically referred to as *quick/slow* and *cocontraction*.

The quick/slow method requires clients to send a quick and strong muscle signal within a certain time frame. For example, if clients reach the preset threshold with their extensor muscle group within the time frame, the wrist may supinate. If their muscle signal does not reach the preset threshold within that time frame, then the terminal device will open. The cocontraction method requires clients to contract both muscles at the same time, also within a certain time frame, to move from component to component (elbow, wrist, or hand). For example, if clients are currently operating their elbow and they want to now operate their hand, they must cocontract both muscles in order to switch to their hand so they may control it. There are other methods to switch between components, although they are less commonly used and typically require more extensive training. Terminal devices, in particular, may have multiple programs to choose from and give clients the option of operating the device the best way that suits their needs (proportional, digital, 1 muscle site or 2 muscle sites). Some terminal devices also have the ability to perform an automatic grasp (detects when a grasped object is slipping and tightens pinch force to avoid losing grasp) or pulsing grasp (unique pulsing for increasing grip force, selectable by digit). It is important for the OT to know how the prosthesis is controlled and which programs are chosen for their clients so they can provide the appropriate training.

Electric terminal devices have been commercially available since the 1960s. The technology remained fairly unchanged until the 1990s with the introduction of proportional control and then in the 2000s with the introduction of multi-articulating hands. Many health care professionals are familiar with the standard tripod grasp that has been used for decades for the grasp and release of objects. Prosthetic manufacturers have recently introduced terminal devices that provide the following:

- Different hand positions
- Flexible wrists
- Digits that move independently
- Individual digits for those missing one or more fingers

With these new components, clients are now able to achieve various hand positions that were not possible before:

- Lateral pinch
- Index point
- Finger abduction/adduction
- Other customizable positions

For those clients who are familiar with the standard tripod pinch technology, these multi-articulating terminal devices may require retraining so they can take full advantage of the new features instead of just relying on the old features. For clients who have not used a previous electric prosthesis, the training may be more straightforward and retraining will not be necessary. Please see the manufacturers' Web sites (see **Table 2**) for more detailed information on specific training tools for their devices. It is also a good idea to get to know your local prosthetic manufacturer representative because they will always have the most up-to-date information.

COMMUNITY REINTEGRATION AND OTHER REFERRALS

In addition to the prosthetic training aspect, the OT should also be involving clients in community-reintegration activities:

- Grocery store runs
- Eating out at a restaurant
- Pumping and paying for gas
- Post office errands
- Working out
- Other daily errands/activities

This practice, with the aid of a skilled health care provider, will provide valuable lessons on how to approach these tasks in a more efficient and body-mechanic-friendly way as well as increase the clients' level of confidence in performing activities on their own. Other areas the OT should address in therapy or by requesting referrals from the physician include, but are not limited to, the following:

- Worksite evaluation
- Home evaluation
- Functional-capacity evaluation or work-hardening evaluation
- Return-to-driving evaluation
- Mental health referrals
- Vocational rehabilitation
- Assistive technology

MULTI-LIMB LOSS

Working with someone who is missing multiple limbs presents unique challenges. There are 6 major points for an OT to keep in mind:

- First, barring any major issues, the longer side is typically treated as the dominant side.
- Second, prosthetic training should begin with the dominant side.
- Third, training should happen one component at a time:
  - Should begin with the terminal device because it is most often used
  - Move on to the next, most-used component (the elbow if transhumeral and the wrist if transradial)
- Fourth, training should progress to the following:
  - Bimanual controls training
  - Repetitive drills
  - Two-handed skill training (see the section on the 3 stages of prosthetic training)
- Fifth, adaptive equipment is a must for someone with bilateral upper limb loss.

Individuals with multi-limb loss should be shown how to accomplish basic self-care tasks with and without their prostheses. In the event they are without their arms for any period of time, it is essential in helping them maintain a certain level of independence. Adaptive equipment will vary from person to person depending on their level of limb loss and desires for independence in the home. For higher levels of limb loss, a helpful chart with adaptive equipment considerations and resources is provided (ie, a dressing tree is extremely beneficial for independence with dressing and don/doff of prostheses or a bidet for independence with toileting) (**Table 3**).

- Sixth and last, a home evaluation is essential to evaluate what areas of the home may need modification in order for clients to be independent with self-care or home-management tasks. Working with a skilled and knowledgeable Americans with Disabilities Act residential contractor is extremely helpful. See **Fig. 5** for a shower set-up example.

Table 3
Bilateral upper limb loss adaptive equipment considerations

ADL Area	Equipment
Toileting	Bidets with wall-mounted control, travel variety, wet wipes, toilet paper on base of toilet
Feeding	U cuffs, swivel utensils, Dycem® (Dycem Ltd, Bristol, UK)
Dressing Prosthetic don/doff	Dressing Tree, industrial strength suction cups with hooks
Grooming, feeding	Goose neck clamps or industrial-strength suction cups with hooks or with adaptive holder on end (hair dryer, razor, deodorant, brushing teeth, suction cup scrub brush, wall-mounted brush)
Communication/computing	Home phone: speakerphone with large buttons Computer, tablet, or smart phone: voice recognition software, mouth stick
Environmental controls	High-technology computerized control: lights, thermostat, kitchen appliances, caregiver call, TV, computer Basic control: mouth stick
Bathing	Wall-mounted sponges, brushes, or soap/shampoo dispenser, handles instead of knobs, pedals for dispensing, prosthetic shower arms, body dryer
Touch screens (phones, tablets, thermostat, kiosks, banking)	Capacitive vs resistive touch screens: specialized gloves (REI/Target), packaged beef jerky, packaged string cheese, specialized stylus, O-Cel-O™ sponge (3M, St. Paul, MN, USA)
Female considerations	Bras, monthly cycles, makeup, hair, shaving legs
Meal preparation	Jar/can opener, paring board, pot/dish holder, dycem, pouring aid, water or beverage dispenser, one-touch storage containers, easy-access condiments
Around the house	Rocker switch lights, handles on doors, swinging doors
Driving	Adapted controls, foot controls or head rest controls for steering, air conditioning/heat, stereo, windows, ignition, horn, wipers, lights, blinkers
Keep in mind preferences, weather/climate	Elastic pants vs jeans, slip-on shoes vs shoelaces, Velcro (Velcro Industries, Manchester, NH) vs buttons or zippers

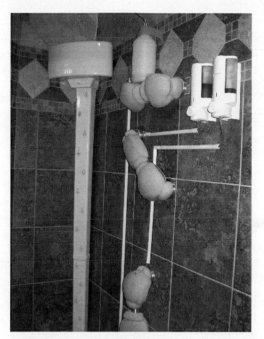

Fig. 5. Bilateral shower setup. (*Courtesy of* Brooke O'Steen, Fort Wayne, IN.)

For those individuals without one or both legs, the adaptive equipment needs and home modifications will vary and be more involved.

OUTCOME MEASURES FROM THE OT'S PERSPECTIVE

There are various standardized tests that OTs use in a clinical setting to document baseline status and progress to prove therapeutic intervention is medically neces- sary. However, many of these commonly used tests are not validated for use with someone who has a prosthesis. Some tests are just not feasible secondary to the length of time to complete and the cost of the test or training to administer the test. Some peer-reviewed articles mention slight modifications to certain tests to accommodate the prosthesis, but these results are not validated and conducted on such a small sample size that it is not meaningful. For more detailed information on the state of upper limb prosthetic outcome measures, please see article by Heinemann and colleagues elsewhere in this issue.

There are 4 outcome measures this OT recommends for use in a clinical setting (see **Table 2**).

1. The Assessment of Capacity for Myoelectric Control
2. Southampton Hand Assessment Procedure
3. Box and Blocks
4. Jebsen Taylor Test of Hand Function

There are many other tests that can also be used depending on what question you are trying to answer and what component of the International Classification of Functioning, Disability, and Health you are addressing (function, activity, participation).

RESOURCES

Typically, an occupational therapy student will spend a few hours in school reading a few pages in a text book about upper limb loss rehabilitation. When practicing OTs do encounter someone missing an arm, they may only see one every few years, which can be attributed to the sheer low numbers of individuals with upper limb loss. This area of rehabilitation for an OT is greatly lacking in continuing education and useful resources. It can become a highly specialized field for an OT who works with these individuals on a regular basis. This OT recommends connecting with prosthetic care facilities experienced in upper limb loss care and prosthetic manufacturers as well as performing thorough Internet searches to learn about conferences, videos, outcome measures, and specific courses related to prosthetic rehabilitation Please see **Table 2** for suggested resources.

TECHNOLOGY: WHAT IS NEW?

Targeted muscle reinnervation (TMR) is a relatively new elective surgery that increases the number of electromyography (EMG) control signals, which in turn has the potential for enhancing prosthetic function. The typical myoelectric prosthesis most OTs are accustomed to have the ability to use up to 2 EMG signals for control. A TMR myoelectric prosthesis has the ability to use up to 6 EMG control signals. The clients with this surgery were seen in research-and-development settings initially for evaluation and testing, but the surgery is now being done worldwide; clients are now being seen in clinical settings with excellent outcomes. An occupational therapy training protocol was developed and is invaluable when working with a TMR client.[7]

Pattern recognition is another recent development in upper limb prosthetics. During the evaluation phase while being hooked up to a group of surface EMG electrodes and computer software, clients will move their phantom limb into a position, for example, hand open, point index finger, elbow flex, wrist supinate, and so forth. The surface electrodes and computer software will pick up a pattern based on what it reads from the group of muscles doing the movements. The various patterns for the different hand and arm movements can be programmed into a client's prosthesis for the prosthetic training phase. The prosthesis may need to be recalibrated every once in awhile, but it is a quick and easy process. The need for 2 or 6 EMG signals is no longer required, which translates to more degrees of freedom and more simultaneous abilities. This innovation is still mostly in the research phase because the commercially available prosthetic hardware is currently not compatible with the pattern-recognition software.

SUMMARY

The prosthetic training process for individuals with upper limb loss can be lengthy; but with a well-designed plan of care, an involved client, early fitting/training, and a collaborative team approach, it can be a very rewarding experience for all parties involved. Rehabilitation will most likely occur in multiple phases over a period of many years because clients will have different ADL needs over time, changes in health can occur, and new componentry is always being developed.

Successful functional outcomes are attainable, and it is important for the OT to manage expectations, seek out available resources, understand the componentry to determine training needs, and continually assess the abilities of clients with upper limb loss to move on to the next stage of skills.

REFERENCES

1. Hubbard S, Galway R, Milner M. The development of myoelectric training methods for pre-school congenital below-elbow amputees and the comparison of two training protocols. J Bone Joint Surg Br 1985;67:273–7.
2. Hermansson L. Structured training of children fitted with myoelectric prostheses. Prosthet Orthot Int 1991;15:88–92.
3. Patton J. Chapter 26: Training the child with a unilateral upper-extremity prosthesis. In: Meier RH, Atkins DJ, editors. Functional restoration of adults & children with upper extremity amputation. New York: Demos Medical Publishing; 2004. p. 297–315.
4. Patton J. Chapter 34D: Upper-limb deficiencies: developmental approach to pediatric upper-limb prosthetic training. In: Bowker HK, Michael JW, editors. Atlas of limb prosthetics: surgical, prosthetic, and rehabilitation principles. 2nd edition. Rosemont (IL): American Academy of Orthopedic Surgeons; 1992. reprinted 2002. p. 779–94.
5. Atkins DJ. Chapter 11: Adult upper limb prosthetic training. In: Bowker HK, Michael JW, editors. Atlas of limb prosthetics: surgical, prosthetic, and rehabilitation principles. 2nd edition. Rosemont (IL): American Academy of Orthopedic Surgeons; 1992. reprinted 2002. p. 277–92.
6. Brenner CD, Brenner JK. The use of preparatory/evaluation/training prostheses in developing evidenced-based practice in upper limb prosthetics. J Prosthet Orthot 2008;20:70–82.
7. Stubblefield KA, Miller LA, Lipschutz RD, et al. Occupational therapy protocol for amputees with targeted muscle reinnervation. J Rehabil Res Dev 2009;46(4): 481–8.

Gait Analysis in Lower-Limb Amputation and Prosthetic Rehabilitation

Alberto Esquenazi, MD

KEYWORDS

- Gait analysis • Lower-limb amputation • Prosthetic rehabilitation • Prosthetic gait

KEY POINTS

- Optimizing the gait characteristics of a person who underwent amputation can enhance the cosmetic qualities of the gait, influence residual limb comfort, and impact the efficiency of ambulation.
- To adequately evaluate the gait characteristics of a person with lower-limb amputation a keen understanding of normal gait, and the possible gait deviations is necessary.
- Biomechanical knowledge of gait and prosthetics is needed to provide optimal clinical care.

Optimizing the gait characteristics of a person who underwent amputation can enhance the cosmetic qualities of the gait pattern; but more importantly, it can also influence residual limb comfort and may affect the efficiency of ambulation and reduce compensatory movements that, over time, may prove damaging to individuals. Gait quality and its velocity can be used as outcome measures in this population.[1–5]

To adequately evaluate the gait characteristics of people with lower-extremity amputations, the clinician must have an understanding of the normal gait as well as the "typical gait deviations" frequently exhibitied by individuals with limb amputation.[6] With this background, specific gait abnormalities can be identified and compared with a catalog of known gait abnormalities to identify the possible contributing factors and available interventions from sound biomechanical knowledge to provide the basis for clinical interventions.[6,7]

The most common cause of an abnormal gait pattern in people with lower-extremity amputations is inadequate prosthetic alignment. The angular and translational position of the socket in relation to the pylon and foot is an important determinant of the walking pattern. Leg length discrepancies, either true or related to a less-than-optimum position of the residual limb within the socket or inefficient suspension, are important secondary causes of gait abnormalities for this population.

Gait and Motion Analysis Laboratory, MossRehab, 60 Township Line Road, Elkins Park, PA 19027, USA
E-mail address: aesquena@einstein.edu

Phys Med Rehabil Clin N Am 25 (2014) 153–167
http://dx.doi.org/10.1016/j.pmr.2013.09.006
1047-9651/14/$ – see front matter © 2014 Elsevier Inc. All rights reserved.

Clinicians who care for individuals with lower-limb amputation must develop a high level of competence in observational gait analysis. Observational gait analysis in a person who underwent amputation is a form of clinical evaluation that requires skill and practice; by observing the motion of the body segments and comparing it with known abnormalities and their underlying mechanisms, one cannot only assume the cause of the abnormal pattern of motion but also develop a corrective strategy and use an iterative process to observe an improvement.

Ultimately, the goal of clinical gait analysis is to optimize the kinematic pattern of the gait so that patients walk as normal as possible. There has been debate in the literature as to whether or not a normal kinematic pattern is necessarily the best or the most efficient gait pattern for individuals with various disabilities; that is, it may be theoretically advantageous for a person who underwent amputation to walk with a kinematic pattern that is different from normal (a compensation) to improve the biomechanical performance of a prosthetic device. Of importance is the desire of many individuals with disabilities, including those with limb amputation, to minimize any external appearances of disability. So even though there may be a metabolic or other disadvantage to a normal-appearing gait, the psychosocial advantages of a normal-appearing gait may far outweigh the relative importance of other considerations.

The human gait is complex, and its fundamental objective is to move safely and efficiently from one point to another. This objective is accomplished by using a cyclical and highly automated movement pattern, with rhythmic, alternating motions of the trunk and extremities that ultimately move the center of mass forward.

Computerized gait analysis involves the reduction of this continuous process into several defined parameters for quantification, evaluation, and comparison. Gait analysis at different times in the rehabilitation process can be useful in the evaluation and optimization of the gait of individuals with lower-limb amputation. In the author's institution, it is particularly helpful in monitoring the progression of rehabilitation; the effectiveness of a particular intervention or for prosthetic component selection; and in the hands of experienced clinicians, for providing detailed information that is useful in the quantification and assessment of prosthetic alignment adjustments with the goal of gait optimization.

NORMAL LOCOMOTION

From a clinical standpoint, it is important to understand the events of the walking cycle. Functional locomotion is concerned with simultaneously solving 5 basic motor problems: (1) the generation of mechanical energy for controlled forward progression, (2) absorption of mechanical energy to minimize shock and/or to decrease the forward progression of the body, (3) the maintenance of a stable upright position, (4) support of the upper body on the lower limb during the stance phase, and (5) control of the lower-extremity position to assure appropriate articulation with the ground during the stance phase and clearance of the foot during the swing phase.

Under normal conditions, comfortable walking speed corresponds to the speed at which the energy cost per unit of distance is minimized. Achievement of energy efficiency depends on unrestricted joint mobility and the precise timing and intensity of muscle action. Abnormal gait biomechanics result in increased energy utilization, usually with a compensatory decrease in walking speed. Often, the compensatory movements necessary for ambulation can produce exaggerated displacements of the center of gravity, which result in increased energy expenditure. Patients with lower limb amputations who have a normal cardiopulmonary mechanism and nutritional status do not ordinarily expend more energy per minute than able-bodied persons, although the energy required per unit distance is increased.

Impaired balance, sensation, and problems with limb clearance can contribute to the anxiety of ambulation and may increase the frequency of loss of balance and falls, a common clinical complaint of this patient population at least in the initial gait-recovery period.

GAIT ANALYSIS

Clinicians routinely do informal, visual analysis of gait in patients with leg amputation. This type of analysis does not provide quantitative information and has many limitations because of the speed and complexity of human locomotion. This circumstance is further complicated by the gait deviations and compensations present in the walking pattern of individuals with lower limb amputation. Gait can be studied through the collection of a wide range of quantitative information in the laboratory using optoelectronic technology and force platforms. In the author's laboratory, they use 3 infrared Coda CX1 (Charnwood Dynamics, Leicester, UK) active marker units and 5 specially designed force platforms (**Fig. 1**). A major advantage provided by these system is the speed of data acquisition and processing, which is essential to allow for the efficient use of the clinician's and patients' time for the effective assessment and intervention of the subject under evaluation. For patients whereby running assessment is the goal, an instrumented treadmill with 2 force platforms that have independent velocity control for each leg is available in highly specialized centers (**Fig. 2**).

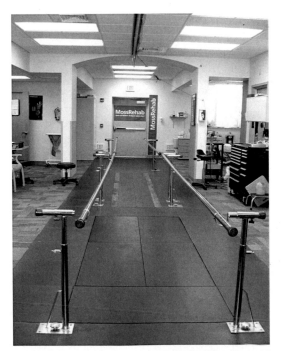

Fig. 1. Gait laboratory with 5 force platforms and removable/adjustable parallel bars.

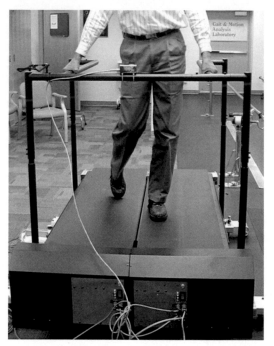

Fig. 2. Instrumented treadmill with 2 force platforms and 2 independent speed-adjustable belts.

KINEMATICS
Temporal and Spatial Descriptive Measures

In order to characterize the gait, basic variables concerning the temporospatial sequencing of stance and swing phases are measured. These parameters are the product of the total integrated walking pattern. A gait analysis report provides calculated data about walking velocity, cadence, stance, and swing times for each limb as well as stride lengths and step lengths usually plotted over comparative gender- and velocity-matched normative data. Theses data also provide measures of symmetry and the impact of interventions on improving the symmetry of walking (**Fig. 3**).

Kinematic data provide a description of movement without regard to the force generating it. The kinematic information is available instantaneously as coordinate data and is processed and displayed as a function of time or, more commonly, as a percent of the gait cycle (normalized). Derived data including joint angles, angular velocities, acceleration, and limb segment rotation are of great utility in the process of gait evaluation. For comparison, velocity-matched normative data with ± 2 SD are plotted (**Fig. 4**).

The magnitude of the ground reaction forces and its relationship to joint centers are the factors that determine moments or torque about a joint, which will indicate the direction and magnitude to generate the kinetic data (**Fig. 5**).

CLINICAL GAIT ANALYSIS IN PEOPLE WITH AMPUTATIONS

Before discussing common gait abnormalities in people with transtibial amputations, it is important to appreciate how their gait patterns differ from normal even under

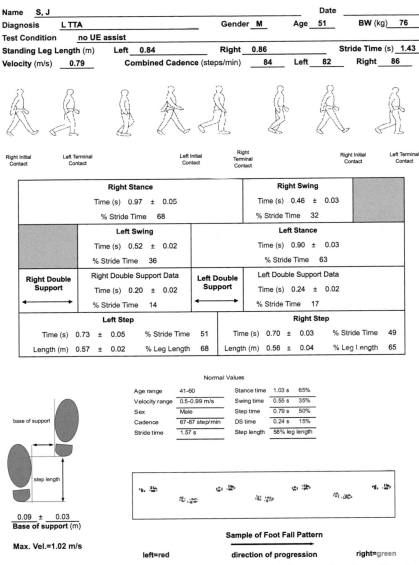

MossRehab   Gait & Motion Analysis Laboratory

Name   S, J _____   Date _____

Diagnosis   **L TTA** _____   Gender **M**   Age **51**   BW (kg) **76**

Test Condition   **no UE assist** _____

Standing Leg Length (m)   Left   **0.84** _____   Right   **0.86** _____   Stride Time (s) **1.43**

Velocity (m/s)   **0.79** _____   Combined Cadence (steps/min)   **84**   Left   **82**   Right   **86**

| Right Initial Contact | Left Terminal Contact | Left Initial Contact | Right Terminal Contact | Right Initial Contact | Left Terminal Contact |

Right Stance	Right Swing	
Time (s) 0.97 ± 0.05	Time (s) 0.46 ± 0.03	
% Stride Time 68	% Stride Time 32	

	Left Swing	Left Stance
	Time (s) 0.52 ± 0.02	Time (s) 0.90 ± 0.03
	% Stride Time 36	% Stride Time 63

Right Double Support	Right Double Support Data	Left Double Support	Left Double Support Data
← →	Time (s) 0.20 ± 0.02	← →	Time (s) 0.24 ± 0.02
	% Stride Time 14		% Stride Time 17

Left Step		Right Step	
Time (s) 0.73 ± 0.05 % Stride Time 51		Time (s) 0.70 ± 0.03 % Stride Time 49	
Length (m) 0.57 ± 0.02 % Leg Length 68		Length (m) 0.56 ± 0.04 % Leg Length 65	

Normal Values

Age range	41-60	Stance time	1.03 s	65%
Velocity range	0.5-0.99 m/s	Swing time	0.55 s	35%
Sex	Male	Step time	0.79 s	50%
Cadence	67-87 step/min	DS time	0.24 s	15%
Stride time	1.57 s	Step length	58% leg length	

base of support

step length

0.09 ±   0.03
Base of support (m)

Max. Vel.=1.02 m/s

Sample of Foot Fall Pattern

left=red   direction of progression   right=green

Fig. 3. Temporal spatial measures of gait with age-matched normative data. (*Courtesy of MossRehab, Einstein Healthcare Network, Philadelphia, PA; with permission.*)

optimum conditions. Firstly, people with transtibial amputations walk more slowly than normal,[8] and their self-selected walking speeds vary with the underlying cause of amputation. In general, the people with traumatic transtibial amputations walk more slowly than age-matched controls, whereas people with dysvascular amputations walk more slowly than people with traumatic amputations.[9,10] The factors that contribute to the slower self-selected gait speed of people with amputations are not known with certainty. Some of the factors that may contribute include the loss of

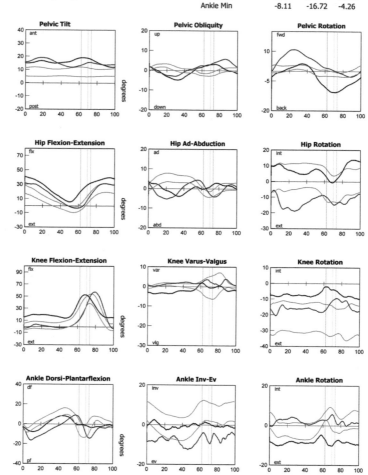

Fig. 4. Kinematic data displayed as a percent of the gait cycle (normalized). Red represents right leg, blue represents left, and gray represents the velocity-matched normative data +/− 1 SD. Vertical line at approximately 70% indicates end of stance and beginning of swing. Data obtained with CODA CX1.

normal sensory motor function in the prosthetic limb with its associated loss of proprioceptive input and balance as well as the loss of normal eccentric controlling and concentric propulsive muscle functions at the foot and ankle. However, most people who have undergone amputation tend to walk at a speed that is concordant with their

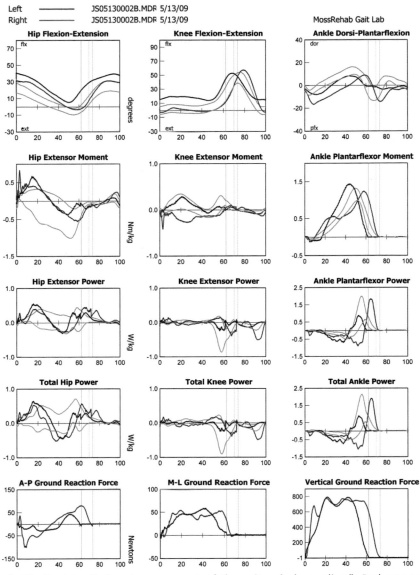

Fig. 5. Kinetic data displayed as a percent of the gait cycle (normalized). Red represents right leg, blue represents left, and gray represents the velocity-matched normative data +/− 1 SD. Vertical line at approximately 70% indicates end of stance and beginning of swing. Data obtained with CODA CX1 and 5 Bertec force platforms (Bertec Corporation, Columbus, OH, USA).

minimum metabolic cost. It may be, therefore, that the slower self-selected walking speed is driven by their desire to walk at the most efficient speed possible, but they may be able to generate higher speeds under special circumstance.

People with amputations also tend to exhibit asymmetries of gait in both stance and swing times between the intact and prosthetic limbs.[6,11] Usually a reduced stance time on the prosthetic limb and a longer step length on the prosthetic limb[11] are present. Shortened stance times on the prosthetic side are also associated with an increased swing time on the prosthetic limb.

The angular kinematics of the lower-extremity joints do also differ between people with amputations and normal subjects. The major differences are at the ankle and knee on the prosthetic side.[8] These differences are largely related to the inability of the prosthetic foot/ankle mechanism to duplicate the normal biomechanical function of the intact musculature, leading to compensatory adaptations in the proximal musculature of the intact and prosthetic limbs.[9,12–14]

Gait Abnormalities in People with Transtibial Amputations

The most easily correctable gait abnormalities seen in people with transtibial amputations are related to leg length discrepancies, prosthetic malalignments, and wearing footwear with heel heights that differ from that used at the time of the initial prosthetic alignment.

Leg length discrepancies

Leg length discrepancies are the common findings and essential to identify because they can result in several adverse effects. Leg length discrepancies in people with amputations can be the result of a prosthesis fabrication error that results in it being either too long or too short, but more commonly it is the result of uncompensated changes in residual limb volume allowing the residual limb to slide in the socket. One of the key reasons prosthetic socks are used in most individuals with transtibial amputations is to compensate for normal changes in residual limb volume. If the residual limb shrinks down, then additional socks should be worn to maintain the optimum position of the residual limb in the socket. If this is not done, the residual limb sinks deeper into the socket resulting in a relatively short prosthetic limb during the stance phase. In contrast, patients who wear too many prosthetic socks or who have an increased residual limb volume relative to the socket resulting from weight gain or fluid accumulation may have a prosthetic leg that is relatively long because the residual limb is out of the socket.

Leg length discrepancies of greater than 2 cm in individuals without amputations lead to an increased metabolic cost of ambulation, increased perceived exertion, and abnormal electromyogram activation during walking.[4]

Leg length discrepancies are noticeable to patients during walking and lead to clinical dissatisfaction because of a perceived limp, at least in individuals with leg length discrepancies resulting from total joint arthroplasty.[15] Although little research has been performed to evaluate the effect of leg length discrepancies in people with amputations, it seems that there is a higher incidence of low back pain in individuals with transfemoral amputations who have a leg length discrepancy.[16]

The most common gait abnormality resulting from a leg prosthetic limb length discrepancy of 2.2 cm or less occurs at the pelvis. Resulting in increased coronal plane pelvic obliquity[17] when the prosthetic limb during double support is about to make floor contact. The pelvic drop on the short side is caused by the need for the limb to reach the ground. Also during the stance phase for the nonamputated limb, midstance knee flexion may be implemented to shorten the longer leg.

In contrast, if the prosthetic limb is long, there may be vaulting on the intact side to increase the prosthetic swing-phase clearance. Vaulting is defined as compensatory active midstance-phase ankle plantarflexion that functionally lengthens the stance-phase limb allowing for more effective contralateral swing-phase clearance of the excessively long prosthetic limb. Another adaptation during the swing phase for an excessively long prosthetic limb is the use of circumduction, which is seen much less commonly in people with transtibial amputations than in people with transfemoral amputations. The implementation of an abducted gait pattern is another adaptation. The difference between a circumducting swing-phase gait and an abducted gait is that in the abducted gait, the limb is in a position of hip abduction throughout both the swing and stance phase, whereas in the circumducted gait, it has a relatively normal position during the stance phase and is brought out into abduction during the swing and then back into a normal coronal plane position before the next succeeding stance phase.

Other deviations frequently encountered are early stance-phase knee flexion or knee hyperextension, which is accompanied by lateral thrust (genu varus). Theses deviations may be the result of a prosthetic foot placed anterior or posterior to its ideal location or the use of a higher or lower heel for the optimal prosthetic alignment (**Fig. 6**).

TRANSFEMORAL PROSTHETIC GAIT DEVIATIONS

In the transfemoral prosthesis, the addition of one intermediate movable knee joint with the potential for additional available prosthetic alignment adjustments complicates the process of understanding the causes and the possible corrections of the gait deviations when compared with the transtibial level prosthesis or the transfemoral prosthesis with a locked knee.

One should avoid the impulse of altering the prosthetic alignment or its components without fully understanding the cause of a deviation and the expected biomechanical effect of an alignment change.

Stance-Phase Problems

One of the most common gait deviations observed in patients with transfemoral amputations is knee flexion during the stance phase; it may result in limb instability, loss

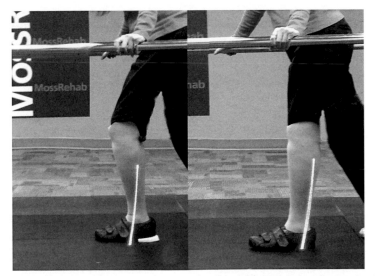

Fig. 6. Depiction of the effect of appropriate heel height (*right*) and higher heel on the prosthetic alignment of a person with transtibial amputation using the forceline visualization system. Note more flexed attitude of the prosthesis for the higher heel.

of standing balance, and falls. Patients are unable to control the knee flexion moment during the stance phase and become fearful of weight bearing on the prosthetic side. This situation results in an inefficient gait pattern that requires the use of upper-limb support or shortening of the step length.

In most cases, prosthetic alignment adjustments to improve knee stability may suffice, but occasionally the use of a mechanical knee brake may be required. The use of a weight-activated locking brake mechanism, polycentric knee, or a hydraulic hinge with or without a microprocessor controller that will allow knee flexion during the swing phase but will prevent accidental knee flexion during the stance phase is desirable over a locked knee. When all of these interventions fail to prevent knee collapse,

A   Gait Analysis Report MossRehab Hospital

Patient Data: PRE

Gender	Age	Date of Birth	Height (m)	Weight (kg)
Male	52	11/56	1.700	76

Gait Parameters	Left	Right
Velocity (m/s)	0.70	0.69
Stride Length (m)	1.03	1.02
Stride Time (s)	1.46	1.48
Step Length (m)	0.56	0.46
Step Time (s)	0.80	0.67
Cadence	75.19	89.15
Percent Stance	62.32	73.36
Swing Time (s)	0.39	0.55
Double Support (s)	0.25	0.28

Joint Angles(deg)	Left	Right	Normal
Hip Range	35.31	35.12	32.98
Hip Max	40.53	31.45	31.09
Hip Min	5.22	-3.67	-1.89
Knee Range	38.73	60.05	49.20
Knee Max	52.64	57.11	54.02
Knee Min	13.91	-2.94	4.82
Ankle Range	16.29	25.56	20.41
Ankle Max	8.18	8.84	16.15
Ankle Min	-8.11	-16.72	-4.26

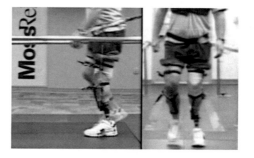

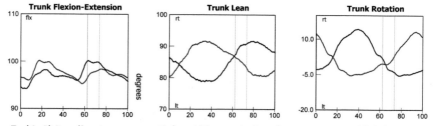

Fig. 7. (*A, B*) Baseline temporospatial and kinematic data from a person with left transtibial amputation displayed as a percent of the gait cycle.

B

Kinematics: Single Cycle

Left	———	JS051
Right	———	JS051
Normal	———	0.4-0.8 m/s

MossRehab Gait Lab

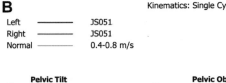

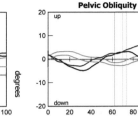

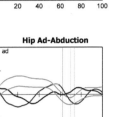

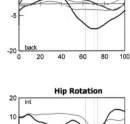

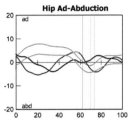

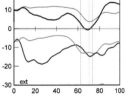

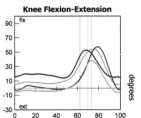

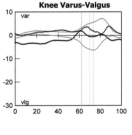

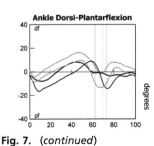

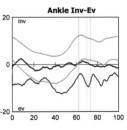

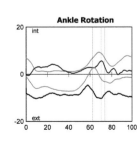

Fig. 7. (*continued*)

only then, a locked knee mechanism should be considered during ambulation. This mechanism will result in a stiff-knee gait pattern during the swing and a lack of knee flexion in early stance phases with the energy-consuming penalty of such deviations and the need of implementing compensations for them.

A   Gait Analysis Report MossRehab Hospital

Patient Data:

Gender	Age	Date of Birth	Height (m)	Weight (kg)
Male	52	11/56	1.700	76

Gait Parameters	Left	Right		Joint Angles(deg)	Left	Right	Normal
Velocity (m/s)	0.83	0.80		Hip Range	39.05	38.02	32.98
Stride Length (m)	1.13	1.13		Hip Max	38.73	33.06	31.09
Stride Time (s)	1.36	1.41		Hip Min	-0.32	-4.96	-1.89
Step Length (m)	0.55	0.58					
Step Time (s)	0.67	0.69		Knee Range	46.00	63.55	49.20
Cadence	89.29	87.46		Knee Max	58.58	59.02	54.02
Percent Stance	65.76	69.65		Knee Min	12.58	-4.53	4.82
Swing Time (s)	0.43	0.47		Ankle Range	15.67	25.26	20.41
Double Support (s)	0.21	0.26		Ankle Max	7.57	6.95	16.15
				Ankle Min	-8.10	-18.31	-4.26

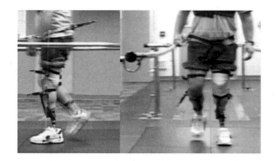

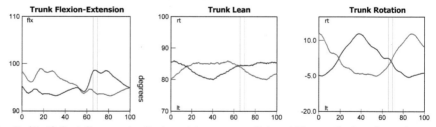

Fig. 8. (*A, B*) Postalignment adjustment temporospatial and kinematic data from the same person. Note improvement in walking velocity and symmetry of the other parameters.

Following are examples of gait changes with different prosthetic alignments in a patient with a left transtibial amputation with gait improvements in velocity, symmetry, and kinematic parameters as documented by 3-dimensional gait analysis.

Note the increase in walking velocity, reduction in trunk lean during the left stance in the postdata photographic image, and the correlated kinematic data reduction in trunk lean and flexion of the patient as well as the improvement toward normalization of the pelvic tilt and rotation, hip flexion extension, and pick ankle motion (**Figs. 7** and **8**).

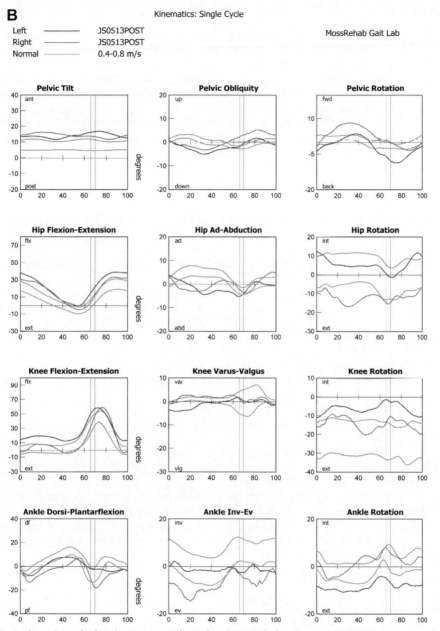

Fig. 8. (*continued*) The data were collected at MossRehab using a CODA CX1 system and 5 Bertec force platforms (Bertec Corporation, Columbus, OH, USA). The data have been normalized and compared with gait velocity, age-matched normative data. The red curves indicate the right leg, blue indicates the left leg, and the gray lines define normal ± 1 SD.

SUMMARY

In summary, gait analysis combined with sound clinical judgment play an important role in elucidating the factors involved in pathologic prosthetic gait and the selection and effects of the available interventions to optimize it.

Detailed clinical evaluation of walking contributes to the analysis of prosthetic gait, but evaluation in the gait laboratory using kinetic and kinematic data is often necessary to quantify and best identify the particular contributions of the multiple variables impacting gait with confidence and assess the results of such intervention. The same approach can be considered when selecting prosthetic components and assessing leg length in this patient population.

REFERENCES

1. Esquenazi A, Keenan MA. Gait analysis. In: Delisa JA, editor. Rehabilitation medicine: principles and practice. 2nd edition. Philadelphia: JB Lippincott; 1991. p. 122–30.
2. Perry J. The use of gait analysis for surgical recommendations in traumatic brain injury. J Head Trauma Rehabil 1999;14(2):116–35.
3. Rosenbaum DA. Human motor control. San Diego (CA): Academic Press; 1991.
4. Treweek SP, Condie ME. Three measures of functional outcome for lower limb amputees: a retrospective view. Prosthet Orthot Int 1998;22:178–85.
5. Winter DA, Sienko SE. Biomechanics of below-knee amputee gait. J Biomech 1988;21:361–7.
6. Esquenazi A. Analysis of prosthetic gait. In: Esquenazi A, editor. Physical medicine and rehabilitation. State of the art reviews, vol. 8, No. 1. Philadelphia: Henley & Belfus, Inc; 1994. p. 201–20.
7. Esquenazi A, Wikoff E, Lucas M. Amputation rehabilitation. In: Grabois M, editor. Physical medicine and rehabilitation -the complete approach. Oxford: Blackwell Science; 2000. p. 1744–60.
8. Segal AD, Orendurff MS, Klute GK, et al. Kinematic and kinetic comparisons of transfemoral amputee gait using C-Leg and Mauch SNS prosthetic knees. J Rehabil Res Dev 2006;43:857–70.
9. Commean PK, Smith KE, Vannier MW. Lower extremity residual limb slippage within the prosthesis. Arch Phys Med Rehabil 1997;78:476–85.
10. Johansson JL, Sherrill DM, Riley PO, et al. A clinical comparison of variable-damping and mechanically passive prosthetic knee devices. Am J Phys Med Rehabil 2005;84:563–75.
11. Powers CM, Rao S, Perry J. Knee kinetics in transtibial amputee gait. Gait Posture 1998;8:1–7.
12. Esquenazi A, DiGiacomo R. Rehabilitation after amputation. J Am Podiatr Med Assoc 2001;91(1):13–22.
13. Wilken JM, Marin R. Gait analysis and training of people with limb loss. In: Loundsbury DE, Lenhart M, editors. Textbooks of military medicine. Washington, DC: Department of the Army, Office of the Surgeon General, Borden Institute; 2010. p. 535–52, Chapter 19.
14. Esquenazi A. Clinical application of joint kinetic analysis in gait. PMR: State of the Art Reviews 2002;16(2):201–14.
15. Sanderson DJ, Martin PE. Lower extremity kinematic and kinetic adaptations in unilateral below-knee amputees during walking. Gait Posture 1997;6:126–36.

16. Esquenazi A, Torres MM. Prosthetic feet and ankle mechanisms. Phys Med Rehabil Clin N Am 1991;2(2):299–309.
17. Kulkarni J, Gaine WJ, Buckley JG, et al. Chronic low back pain in traumatic lower limb amputees. Clin Rehabil 2005;19(1):81–6.

Complications Following an Amputation

Stanley Yoo, MD

KEYWORDS

- Upper limb amputation • Lower limb amputation • Diabetes • Vascular disease
- Trauma

KEY POINTS

- There are numerous complications of amputation that make comprehensive rehabilitation management of the patient with amputation a challenging task.
- Optimal management comes from a coordinated, multidisciplinary approach in which each specialty has a specific and indispensable role in improving acute issues and the prevention or improvement of long-term, adverse sequelae.
- In addition to improving functional mobility and independence, physical and occupational therapists are pivotal in the evaluation and management of phantom pain, residual limb pain, and secondary musculoskeletal complaints and overuse syndromes.
- Meanwhile psychology and recreational therapists can provide the patient with resources and strategies to manage the mood disorders that could otherwise negatively impact the patient's functional outcome.
- Recreational therapists, in conjunction with physical and occupational therapists, also play an important role in developing strategies for successful reintegration into society and life roles.

INTRODUCTION

In 2005 there were an estimated 1.6 million individuals in the United States living with limb loss. This number has been projected to more than double by 2050 to 3.6 million,[1] making an understanding of management of the individual with amputation essential for the physiatrist. In developed nations, disease is the leading cause for amputation, with the incidence of major amputation in patients with diabetes being approximately 10-fold that of nondiabetic dysvascular patients in certain populations.[2] As such, many of the complications after amputation may, in fact, be attributable to the underlying disease process and not dissimilar to issues that led to the initial amputation. Other complications are potential sequelae of amputations of nearly any cause.

The author does not have any relationship to disclose with any company that has a direct financial interest in the subject matter or materials discussed in this article.
Moss Rehab, 60 Township Line Road, Elkins Park, PA 19027, USA
E-mail address: skyoo13@yahoo.com

Phys Med Rehabil Clin N Am 25 (2014) 169–178
http://dx.doi.org/10.1016/j.pmr.2013.09.003
1047-9651/14/$ – see front matter © 2014 Elsevier Inc. All rights reserved.

Treatment, therefore, may not vary significantly among different amputation populations. This article highlights common complications after amputation and discusses management strategies for each. As with many disease processes, the multidisciplinary approach with coordination of care among the physiatrist, therapists, nursing staff, psychologist, and other specialists proves to be most effective and rewarding in optimal management of patients with amputation.

MUSCULOSKELETAL COMPLICATIONS

It is estimated that 20% of people with amputation underwent amputation early in life,[3] and therefore, may have to deal with the adverse sequelae of long-term altered postural and gait mechanics, relative inactivity, muscular imbalances, and surgical complications. These complications include joint contracture, early degenerative joint disease and overuse injury on the intact limb, back pain, osteopenia/osteoporosis, fracture, and disuse atrophy. Many of these complications can be avoided with diligent care and patient education, which should begin immediately in the postoperative period, and be carried over into the remainder of the patient's life.

Joint contracture is a common occurrence after lower limb amputation for multiple reasons, with many patients with transtibial amputation developing knee flexion contracture and/or hip flexion contracture, and those with transfemoral amputation developing hip flexion and abduction contracture. First, because patients are generally less active immediately after their amputations and spend most of their time resting in either a seated or a lying position, it is easy for hip and knee flexion contractures to develop because there are very few resting postures where these joint are positioned in anything other than the flexed position. Second, the muscle imbalance created by the amputation itself can predispose the involved joint to developing contracture. It has been found that cleaved muscles after transfemoral amputation can atrophy 40% to 60%, while intact muscle in the amputated limb can still atrophy up to 30%.[4] Loss of hip adductor strength can predispose to hip abduction contracture, while avoiding fixation of the iliotibial tract in an attempt to prevent hip abduction contracture can predispose to hip flexion contracture as the hip extension torque of the gluteus maximus is decreased.

Both performing and instructing the patient in range-of-motion exercises is paramount in re-creating a natural and efficient gait pattern, and prevention of skin breakdown as well as pain in the prosthesis. For the patient with transtibial amputation, the prescription of a residual limb support allows the knee of the amputated limb to be positioned in extension while the patient is seated in his or her wheelchair. Immediate postoperative rigid dressings (IPORD), immediate postoperative prostheses (IPOP), as well as bi-valved casts can aid in prevention of joint contracture and have the added advantages of protecting the operative wound and controlling postoperative limb swelling. However, they require both skill and time to create, need to be remade as the limb reduces in size, and in the case of the IPORD and IPOP, do not allow for easy viewing of the surgical incision. Once contracture has already developed, serial casting may be used to stretch the joint, while those cases refractory to conservative measures may require surgical management.

Altered gait and postural patterns in the lower limb amputee can come from learned walking patterns to compensate for weakness, joint contracture, a sensation of instability, improper prosthetic fit, or from any combination of the above. Up to 23% difference in ground reaction force has been found between the intact and amputated limb, and persons with amputation also typically spend more time on their intact limb. With increased forces on the joints of the intact limb there is a greater prevalence of knee pain and radiographic evidence of patellofemoral osteoarthritis in the intact limb.[3] Asymmetry in gait and increased dependence on proximal musculature have also been associated with a 3- to 6-fold incidence of osteoarthritis of both hips in patients with lower limb amputation, with a nearly 3-fold incidence of hip osteoarthritis in the amputated as compared with the intact limb, while decreased forces through the prosthetic limb may contribute to osteoporosis/osteopenia and fracture due to low bone mineral density. With respect to low back pain, hip flexion contracture requires hyperlordosis of the lumbosacral spine to maintain upright posture and may cause or exacerbate preexisting low back pain. Similarly, limb length asymmetry due to suboptimal prosthetic fitting or inadequate fit within the prosthetic socket can also cause gait and postural asymmetry as well as pain by increasing the lateral tilt of the pelvis in the frontal plane, and therefore, requiring a compensatory scoliosis.

Overuse of the intact limb in upper limb amputees is also associated with a higher incidence of self-reported musculoskeletal pain in the upper limb amputee. Common areas of pain in the upper limb amputee were in the neck/upper back (57%) and shoulders (58.9%). Interestingly, prosthesis wear was not found to affect this pain.[5]

In addition to range-of-motion exercises, particular attention should be paid to strengthening, not only of the proximal muscles of the amputated limb, but also of the intact limb. In the patient with transtibial amputation, knee and hip extensor strength is essential for maintaining knee stability during stance, while in those with transfemoral amputation focus should be placed on hip girdle and core strengthening. It is equally important to coach patients on proper gait mechanics, focusing on establishing symmetry in stance times and step lengths between the intact and amputated limbs and avoiding unnecessary compensatory strategies, which may prove to be energy costly and cause undue stresses to muscles and joints of the intact limb. Finally, fit and alignment should be optimized to ensure proper standing and walking posture and limb length symmetry (in patients with preexisting limb length asymmetry, this may not be warranted because matching limb lengths may, in fact, prove uncomfortable due anatomic and postural compensations made over time). For the patient with upper limb amputation, focus should be placed on shoulder girdle strengthening and scaption exercises, as these motions are frequently used for control of the upper limb prosthesis, particularly in body-powered designs.

Heterotopic ossification seems to be a common occurrence, particularly after traumatic amputation where the amputation site occurs within the initial zone of injury.[6] However, not all instances are problematic. Those that are may be treated conservatively with adjustments to the prosthetic socket to provide pressure relief to the area of bony prominence. Approximately 80% of patients with radiographic evidence were found to either be asymptomatic or able to be managed successfully nonoperatively. For cases refractory to conservative measures, surgical excision can be performed with good success rates.

DERMATOLOGIC CONSIDERATIONS

Disruption of skin integrity is a major causative factor for amputation, especially in patients with diabetes. Likewise, patients with amputation may be at increased risk for revision amputation or amputation of the contralateral limb if the protective barrier offered by the skin is not maintained. Up to 41% of persons with lower limb amputation experience skin problems on their residual limb,[7] with the most commonly reported issues being wounds, abscesses, and blisters. Dermatologic issues may be secondary to surgical complications, repetitive injury, or reaction to occlusion of the skin. Wound dehiscence is a major complication that requires immediate referral back to the surgeon. Wound dehiscence most commonly occurs from local trauma to the area of the healing surgical incision. Care must be taken to avoid trauma or distraction of the skin edges as the wound heals. In a patient demonstrating impulsive or unsafe behavior, the incision may be protected by the fabrication of an IPORD/IPOP or a bivalve cast. A bivalve cast also may offer a measure of comfort to patients whose anxiety about their healing limb limits their ability to perform transfers or activities of daily living independently. Residual limb shaping begins shortly after amputation to control postoperative swelling and prepare the limb for eventual fitting with a prosthesis. Until enough healing has occurred for wound closure with either staples or sutures to be safely removed, the application of a residual limb shrinker is avoided, because shear forces from the shrinker could pull apart the healing skin edges and either prevent wound healing or dehisce the wound. Once wound closure devices are removed, application of a shrinker is generally considered safe. Sutures or staples are generally maintained longer in patients with diabetes, given their predisposition to a more protracted wound healing course.

The skin of the residual limb should be monitored closely by both the clinician and the patient, especially in the prosthetic training period, as excessive pressure or shear within the prosthetic socket can very quickly lead to skin breakdown. These pressures can be caused by suboptimal socket fit and/or prosthetic alignment, and therefore, the patient must be observed during gait and standing (for lower limb amputees) as well as at the time of donning. A discussion of specific gait deviations and prosthetic alignment is beyond the scope of this article, but knowledge of how each deviation may cause skin breakdown and how to correct it is important in prosthetic management. Generally speaking, socket fit should allow for displacement of pressure over a greater surface area, taking care to offload pressure from intolerant areas (eg, hamstrings, tibial crest, tibial tuberosity) and preferentially load more tolerant areas (popliteal area, patellar tendon). It is a common misconception among patients that padding should be added to areas of soreness. Adding padding to areas of excessive pressure will only serve to increase focal pressure and increase the risk of skin breakdown. Instead, padding should be added around the area of pressure (eg, "keying in" the tibial crest by placing padding medial and lateral to it) to offload the area of prominence successfully.

Dermatologic conditions related to occlusion can be challenging to manage, because in the patient using a prosthesis, much of the day is spent with the residual limb covered. Hyperhidrosis is a common complaint with prosthetic wear (23%–70% of amputees[8,9]) and can become problematic if persistent maceration of the skin causes breakdown. Conservative treatments include use of either an over-the-counter or prescription medication, changing from a nonbreathable gel liner and suspension system to a more breathable system (eg, changing from a total surface bearing socket with gel liner to a patellar tendon bearing socket with a pelite insert). Botulinum toxin has been shown to have good effect for hyperhidrosis refractory to the above management strategies.[10,11] Skin eruptions (eg, folliculitis) can be reduced with optimal skin hygiene and liner care.[8] Daily washing of the residual limb with mild soap and water is recommended, and daily cleaning can be performed with either mild soap and water or alcohol, depending on the liner type. For those patients in whom inflammation has developed into superficial abscess, incision and drainage and treatment with antibiotics are warranted. Dermatitis may be a response to the liner material and may warrant changing the type of liner used; however, anecdotally, use of an antihistamine cream has offered relief to some patients who have experienced pruritus without erythema or other evidence of frank contact dermatitis.

Monitoring of skin on the intact limb is equally important to skin care for the residual limb. In the dysvascular patient with diabetes, xeroderma, or dry skin, is a common occurrence because of impairment of cutaneous glands. Care should be taken to keep the skin adequately moisturized in areas that tend to get dry easily (eg, the lower legs), whereas areas prone to maceration (eg, between the toes) should be kept dry with the use of material such as lambs wool, which serves to ventilate and dry out the skin. Regular skin hygiene and skin checks should be used to maintain skin integrity. Maintaining skin integrity may be difficult for the patient with impaired mobility and flexibility or impaired vision (eg, the patient with diabetic retinopathy). Skin checks can be facilitated with the use of long-handled mirrors, with digital pictures from a camera phone, or by training a caregiver in proper skin inspection. As excessive shear and pressure from the prosthetic socket can cause callusing and breakdown, so can improperly fitting shoe wear on the intact foot. Shoes with an accommodating toe box help to reduce pressure and callusing over bony prominences, while pressure relieving buildups (eg, metatarsal bars/pads) and toe rockers may be necessary to reduce local pressures in the foot for those with joint motion restriction. Orthopedic or "diabetic" shoes generally do very well at accomplishing adequate pressure relief, but are often cost prohibitive if not covered by insurance. In these instances, it is recommended that the patient buy shoes from a specialty shoe store, where sales representatives are generally more knowledgeable and may aid in making the appropriate foot wear choice.

PAIN

Statistics vary considerably regarding the prevalence of pain in patients with amputation, in part due to study methods and also in part due to the difficulty in characterizing the different types of pain experienced by persons with amputation. Nonetheless, pain is a significant cause for morbidity in the immediate postoperative period as well as long term. Phantom limb pain (PLP) is defined as painful sensations perceived in the missing limb after amputation, while residual limb pain (RLP) is perceived as originating in the residual portion of the limb (ie, the stump).[12] Estimates have placed the prevalence of PLP anywhere from a more conservative 40% to as high as 85%,[13] while RLP was similarly widely variable with estimates of chronic RLP ranging from 10% to 74%. Complicating the pain assessment is that RLP, while all occurring in the same general area, can vary in character (burning vs shocklike, aching, throbbing) as well as cause. The prevalence of pain in areas other than around the site of amputation is also high, with chronic back pain being a complaint in 52% of both upper and lower limb amputees, neck pain in 31% of lower limb amputees and 43% of upper limb amputees, and contralateral limb pain present in 33% and 43% of unilateral upper and lower limb amputees, respectively.[13,14] These secondary areas of pain are likely, in large part, attributable to overuse syndromes and compensatory strategies and are discussed above.

It has long been postulated that both central and peripheral factors as well as psychological factors have a role in PLP. Understanding proven as well as postulated mechanisms for the generation of PLP allows for an understanding of common pharmacologic and nonpharmacologic treatment strategies that are currently being used and investigated. Centrally, deafferentation of the somatosensory cortex, as occurs with amputation, has been shown on functional magnetic resonance imaging to be followed by cortical reorganization, in which the representation of adjacent body structures invades that of the missing limb (eg, the cortical representation of the face invading the representation of the amputated hand).[15] In the case of the amputated hand, it was found in one study that facial gestures (lip pursing) would activate not only bilateral M1 and S1 lip face areas of the cortex, but also the contralateral M1, and to a lesser extent, S1 areas of the hand. There was also evidence that the opposite occurred, where there was expansion of the area of activation for the missing limb to adjacent structures, so that activation of the hand would also cause a similar activation in the facial somatosensory cortex. Other areas of activation included bilateral insula, anterior cingulate cortex, thalamus, and cerebellum.

In this study, patients underwent mental imagery therapy, in which a combination of the body-scan exercise and imagined movement of and sensation in the phantom limb were used. In the body scan exercise, patients learned to concentrate on sensations from each area of the body consecutively, including the phantom arm and hand. Once a state of relaxation was achieved, the recruit was encouraged to imagine comfortable and thorough movement and sensation in the phantom limb. After completing this intervention, there was an overall decrease in phantom limb pain, and repeated functional magnetic resonance imaging studies also showed there was no longer activation of the hand area of the somatosensory cortex with the lip pursing activity, nor was there activation of the facial somatosensory cortex with imagined movement of the amputated hand.

It is unclear as to why the deafferentation and subsequent expansion of the cortical representation of adjacent structures that occurs with cortical reorganization cause pain, but a proposed mechanism is that unopposed motor efferent signals without a corresponding inhibitory afferent sensory signal that the task is complete may incite the dysesthesia.[16] Another thought is that there is a network of neurons, or "neuromatrix," spanning several different areas of the brain (eg, thalamus, somatosensory cortex, limbic system)[17] that create a neurosignature, which is the basis for the sensation of self. When there is abnormal sensory input, as the case would be with amputation, the neurosignature changes, causing the phantom pain. Although these theories remain difficult to prove, altering these reorganizational central changes is the basis for several nonpharmacalogic interventions.

Aside from mental imagery, mirror therapy has also shown promise in altering cortical reorganization for the benefit of decreasing phantom pain. Ramachandran and Rogers-Ramachandran[18] described the use of mirrors to reflect the image of the intact limb, giving the appearance of 2 intact limbs. One study showed improvement in all subjects performing mirror therapy, whereas those subjects in groups performing mental imagery or in which the mirror was covered did not experience similar benefit or even experienced worsening of their pain.[19] Interestingly, when the remaining 2 groups crossed over and initiated mirror therapy, their phantom pain similarly improved. Another case report demonstrated a dose-dependent improvement in phantom pain in one individual, with complete resolution of phantom pain with daily self-administered mirror therapy.[20]

The proposed mechanisms of spinal involvement in phantom pain are largely speculative, based on anecdotal evidence and animal studies. Theories include overactive peripheral nerve signals causing central sensitization,[21] by effecting synaptic changes to the dorsal horn neurons and making them hyperexcitable. Low threshold afferents may be linked to neurons carrying nociceptive input, or inhibitory neurons may be destroyed by rapid discharge from injured tissue, causing the spinal cord to be hyperexcitable. Another thought is that deafferentation leads to a general disinhibition of the spinal cord with reduction in GABAergic activity and opioid receptors. Nevertheless, another mechanism, like in the cortex, may be a local reorganization of regions of the spinal cord in which the deafferentated limb was originally represented.[22]

Because there are numerous proposed central, peripheral, and psychological mechanisms to PLP, the approach to pharmacologic treatment of PLP is fairly similar to that of other forms of neuropathic pain. Although tricycyclic antidepressants and sodium channel blockers have been listed as treatments of choice for neuropathic pain,[23] gapapentin and newer classes of antidepressants are commonly used as well as calcium channel blockers and muscle relaxants. In the early postoperative period as well as in chronic phantom pain, several interventions have been attempted including epidural injection, regional nerve blocks, calcitonin, and mechanical vibratory stimulation in an effort to prevent central sensitization phenomenon. However, a review of trials using these interventions has yet to provide conclusive support for any of these treatments.[24,25] Similarly, although transcutaneous electrical nerves stimulation is commonly used in the treatment of PLP, there have been no large multicenter randomized control trials confirming the efficacy of this modality, and the evidence behind its use remains largely anecdotal.

RLP must be assessed critically, because the character and nature of the pain may give clues as to the cause. As previously alluded to, musculoskeletal complaints in an individual who is using a prosthesis should prompt an investigation into the appropriateness of the alignment and socket fit, limb length, and any concerns regarding overuse injury should be addressed. Burning and shocklike dysesthesias may be treated with a similar pharmacologic as that used for PLP, although dysesthesias elicited with palpation over the residual limb may indicate neuroma. In the case of neuroma, treatment may begin with pressure relief within the prosthetic socket or simple avoidance of exposure to pressure. Local neuroma injection with steroid and lidocaine may be attempted as well. Symptoms such as claudication, or pain in association with erythema, drainage, fever, or pain out of proportion to physical examination findings may warrant further investigation with studies or imaging to rule out vascular compromise and infection of either the bone or the soft tissue. Pending study results, a surgical evaluation may be necessary.

It must be remembered that there is a significant psychological component to perception of pain, including PLP and RLP. An association between stress and the onset and exacerbation of PLP has been shown,[26] and, not surprisingly, in patients with poor coping strategies, pain was found to be more disruptive to daily life than in those who demonstrate good coping skills.[27] It has been the experience of this author that relief of PLP is optimally achieved when a multidisciplinary approach is taken, combining pharmacologic management with modalities, patient education, and interventions when necessary. Mirror therapy and mental imagery techniques have been taught by physical/occupational therapists and psychologists alike, while breathing and coping strategies can be reviewed by both psychologists and recreational therapists. When possible, coordination of care and open communication among all specialties, as is possible with a dedicated multidisciplinary amputee program, enables clinicians to determine the proper combination of treatments to treat the patient most effectively.

PSYCHIATRIC CONSIDERATIONS

Limb loss is found to be associated with psychiatric conditions, which have been shown to have a negative impact on rehabilitative outcomes in chronic conditions.[28,29] Depression is a major comorbidity among patients with amputation, with prevalence rates between 28% and 42%[30-32] as compared with 5.4% in the general population.[33] Further evaluation shows prevalence of major depressive disorder to be higher in those experiencing limb loss due to disease (eg, diabetes, vascular disease, tumor) at 51.4% than those experiencing traumatic limb loss (34.7%).[31] These statistics are of specific significance in developed nations, where the overwhelming cause for amputation is disease. Furthermore, it is estimated that 42% of those with depressive symptoms reported an unmet need for mental health services.[32] There is also a significantly high rate for acute stress disorder and posttraumatic stress disorder in the setting of traumatic amputation, with prevalence of posttraumatic stress disorder reported at between 33% and 72%.[34,35] The high prevalence of coexisting psychiatric conditions highlights the need for concomitant psychiatric support both immediately after amputation and long term, to maximize rehabilitative outcomes and successful reintegration of patients into community and life roles.

SUMMARY

There are numerous complications of amputation that make comprehensive rehabilitation management of the patient with amputation a challenging task. Optimal management comes from a coordinated, multidisciplinary approach in which each specialty has a specific and indispensable role in improving acute issues and the prevention or improvement of long-term, adverse sequelae. In addition to improving functional mobility and independence, physical and occupational therapists are pivotal in the evaluation and management of phantom pain, RLP, and secondary musculoskeletal complaints and overuse syndromes. In the case of the prosthetic user, this is done in conjunction with the prosthetist, who ensures the proper fit and alignment and assists in the selection of appropriate componentry for the patient. Meanwhile psychology and recreational therapists can provide the patient with resources and strategies to manage the mood disorders that could otherwise negatively impact the patient's functional outcome. Recreational therapists, in conjunction with physical and occupational therapists, also play an important role in developing strategies for successful reintegration into society and life roles. Finally, the rehabilitation physician is responsible for and coordinates the care of all specialties, providing pharmacologic and/or interventional management of symptoms when necessary, prescribing the prosthesis, and referring to other specialists when appropriate.

REFERENCES

1. Ziegler-Graham K, MacKenzie E, Ephraim PL, et al. Estimating the prevalence of limb loss in the United States: 2005 to 2050. Arch Phys Med Rehabil 2008;89: 422–9.
2. Moxey PW, Gogalniceanu P, Hinchliffe RJ, et al. Lower extremity amputation: a review of global variability incidence. Diabet Med 2011;28:1144–53.
3. Gailey R, Allen K, Castles J, et al. Review of secondary physical conditions associated with lower-limb amputation and long-term prosthesis use. J Rehabil Res Dev 2008;45(1):15–29.
4. Jaegers MH, Arendzen JH, de Jongh HJ. Changes in hip musculature after above knee amputation. Clin Orthop Relat Res 1995;319:276–84.
5. Ostlie K, Franklin RJ, Skjeldal OH, et al. Musculoskeletal pain and overuse syndromes in adult acquired major upper-limb amputees. Arch Phys Med Rehabil 2011;92(12):1967–73.
6. Potter BK, Burns TC, Lacap AP, et al. Heterotopic ossification following traumatic and combat-related amputations: prevalence, risk factors, and preliminary results of excision. J Bone Joint Surg Am 2007;89(3):476–86.
7. Bui KM, Raugi GJ, Nguyen VQ, et al. Skin problems in individuals with lower-limb loss: literature review and proposed classification system. J Rehabil Res Dev 2009;46(9):1085–90.
8. Hachisuka K, Nakamura T, Ohmine S, et al. Hygiene problems of residual limb and silicone liners in transtibial amputees wearing the total surface bearing socket. Arch Phys Med Rehabil 2001;82:1286–90.

9. Dillingham TR, Pezzin LE, MacKenzie EJ, et al. Use and satisfaction with prosthetic devices among persons with trauma-related amputations: a long term outcome study. Am J Phys Med Rehabil 2001;80:563–71.

10. Kern U, Kohl M, Seifert U, et al. Botulinum toxin type B in the treatment of residual limb hyperhidrosis for lower limb amputees. Am J Phys Med Rehabil 2011;90(4): 321–9.

11. Charrow A, DiFazio M, Foster L, et al. Intradermal botulinum toxin type A injection effectively reduces residual limb hyperhidrosis in amputees: a case series. Arch Phys Med Rehabil 2008;89:1407–9.

12. Davis RW. Phantom sensation, phantom pain, and stump pain. Arch Phys Med Rehabil 1993;74:79–91.

13. Ehde DM, Czerniecki JM, Smith DG, et al. Chronic phantom sensations, phantom pain, residual limb pain, and other regional pain after lower limb amputation. Arch Phys Med Rehabil 2000;81:1038–44.

14. Hanley MA, Ehde DM, Jensen M, et al. Chronic pain associated with upper-limb loss. Am J Phys Med Rehabil 2009;88(9):742–51.

15. MacIver K, Lloyd DM, Kelly S, et al. Phantom limb pain, cortical reorganization and the therapeutic effect of mental imagery. Brain 2008;131:2181–91.

16. Harris JA. Cortical origin of pathological pain. Lancet 1999;354:1464–6.

17. Melzack RA. Phantom limbs and the concept of a neuromatrix. Trends Neurosci 1990;13:88–92.

18. Ramachandran VS, Rogers-Ramachandran D. Synaesthesia in phantom limbs induced with mirrors. Proc Biol Sci 1996;263:377–86.

19. Chan BL, Wit R, Charrow AP, et al. Mirror therapy for phantom limb pain. N Engl J Med 2007;357:2206–7.

20. Darnall BD. Self-delivered home-based mirror therapy for lower limb phantom pain. Am J Phys Med Rehabil 2009;88(1):78–81.

21. Doubell TP, Mannion RJ, Woolf CJ. The dorsal horn: state-dependent sensory processing, plasticity and the generation of pain. In: Wall PD, Melzack RA, editors. Textbook of pain. 4th edition. Edinburgh (United Kingdom): Churchill Livingstone; 1999. p. 165–81.

22. Flor H. Phantom-limb pain: characteristics, causes, and treatment. Lancet Neurol 2002;1:182–9.

23. Sindrup SH, Jensen TS. Efficacy of pharmacological treatments of neuropathic pain: an update and effect related to mechanism of drug action. Pain 1999;83: 389–400.

24. Halbert J, Crotty M, Cameron ID. Evidence for the optima management of acute and chronic phantom pain: a systematic review. Clin J Pain 2002; 18(2):84–92.

25. Mulvey MR, Bagnall AM, Johnson MI, et al. Transcutaneous electrical nerve stimulation for phantom pain and stump pain following amputation in adults. Cochrane Pain, Palliative Care and Supportive Care Group. Cochrane Database Syst Rev 2013;(4):CD007264.

26. Arena JG, Sherman RA, Bruno GM, et al. The relationship between situational stress and phantom limb pain: cross-lagged correlational data from six month pain logs. J Psychosom Res 1990;34:71–7.

27. Hill A, Niven CA, Knussen C. The role of coping in adjustment to phantom limb pain. Pain 1995;62:79–86.

28. Ciechanowski PS, Katon WJ, Russo JE, et al. The relationship of depressive symptoms to symptom reporting, self-care and glucose control in diabetes. Gen Hosp Psychiatry 2003;25:246–52.

29. Felker B, Katon W, Hedrick SC, et al. The association between depressive symptoms and health status in patients with chronic pulmonary disease. Gen Hosp Psychiatry 2001;23:56–61.

30. Kashani JH, Frank RG, Kashani SR, et al. Depression among amputees. J Clin Psychiatry 1983;44:256–8.

31. Cansever A, Uzun O, Yildiz C, et al. Depression in men with traumatic lower part amputation: a comparison to men with surgical lower part amputation. Mil Med 2003;168:106–9.

32. Darnall BD, Epharim P, Wegener ST, et al. Depressive symptoms and mental health service utilization among persons with limb loss: results of a national survey. Arch Phys Med Rehabil 2005;86:650–8.

33. Pratt LA, Brody DJ. Depression in the United States household population, 2005–2006. NCHS Data Brief 2008;(7):1–8.

34. Copuroglu C, Ozcan M, Yilmaz B, et al. Acute stress disorder and post-traumatic stress disorder following traumatic amputation. Acta Orthop Belg 2010;76(1): 90–3.

35. Abeyasighe NL, de Zoysa P, Bandara KM, et al. The prevalence of symptoms of post-traumatic stress disorder among soldiers with amputation of a limb or spinal cord injury: a report from a rehabilitation centre in Sri Lanka. Psychol Health Med 2012;17(3):376–81.

Outcome Instruments for Prosthetics: Clinical Applications

Allen W. Heinemann, PhD[a,b,*], Lauri Connelly, OTR/L[a],
Linda Ehrlich-Jones, PhD, RN[a,b], Stefania Fatone, PhD, BPO[b]

KEYWORDS

- Artificial limbs • Amputation • Assessment of patient outcomes
- Outcome and process assessment (health care) • Prostheses • Treatment outcome

KEY POINTS

- Accreditors expect prosthetists to monitor patient outcomes as part of routine clinical practice.
- Outcomes of patient care can be performance-based or reported by patients.
- Important aspects of care to be monitored include mobility, functional status, quality of life, and satisfaction with services.
- Instruments may be developed specifically for adults with amputations or for general populations; several general-purpose instruments are suitable for adults with amputations.
- Routine monitoring of outcomes allows clinicians to address patient concerns in a timely manner and to implement quality-improvement initiatives while fulfilling accreditation requirements.
- Emerging information about responsiveness of outcome measures improves their clinical utility.

INTRODUCTION: NATURE OF THE PROBLEM

The American Board for Certification in Prosthetics, Orthotics and Pedorthics (ABC) accreditation standards are designed to enhance the quality of health care in prosthetic and orthotic practice, and to help increase efficiency and support initiatives that improve patient outcomes. Facility accreditation helps ABC achieve specific

Funding: This research was funded by the National Institute on Disability and Rehabilitation Research (NIDRR) of the US Department of Education under Grant No. H133E080009 (Principal Investigators: Steven Gard and Stefania Fatone). The opinions contained in this publication are those of the grantee and do not necessarily reflect those of the Department of Education.

[a] Center for Rehabilitation Outcomes Research, Rehabilitation Institute of Chicago, 345 E Superior Street, Chicago, IL 60611, USA; [b] Department of Physical Medicine and Rehabilitation, Feinberg School of Medicine, Northwestern University, 710 North Lake Shore Drive, #1022, Chicago, IL 60611, USA
* Corresponding author. Center for Rehabilitation Outcomes, Research, Rehabilitation Institute of Chicago, 345 E Superior Street, Chicago, IL 60611.
E-mail address: a-heinemann@northwestern.edu

Phys Med Rehabil Clin N Am 25 (2014) 179–198
http://dx.doi.org/10.1016/j.pmr.2013.09.002
1047-9651/14/$ – see front matter © 2014 Elsevier Inc. All rights reserved.

goals, including promoting the welfare of persons with disabilities by establishing standards for those engaged in the fitting of prostheses and orthoses. ABC defines 6 categories of standards including quality assessment and improvement. However, provider enthusiasm for quality improvement through routine outcomes monitoring is diminished by the time and expense required as well as limitations in the psychometric properties of many instruments, in particular the validation of generic instruments with prosthesis users, availability of norms, and evidence of responsiveness or sensitivity of measures to change. This review is designed to provide up-to-date information on the psychometric properties of outcome instruments, allowing prosthetists to select instruments to improve the quality of their services.

In recent years, the American Academy of Orthotists and Prosthetists (AAOP) have published findings from a series of state-of-the-science conferences, 2 of which address lower and upper limb prosthetic outcome instruments. The review of lower limb prosthetic outcome measures by Condie and collegues[1] identified 25 instruments that assess mobility, function, and quality of life. Wright's[2] review of upper limb prosthetic outcome measures identified 7 outcome measures for adults in 4 categories: hand function, upper limb functional abilities, overall functional abilities and participation, and quality of life.

Several other recent reviews of lower and upper limb outcome measures for prosthesis users have been organized using the International Classification of Functioning, Disability and Health (ICF). Hebert and colleagues[3] reviewed measures of body function applicable to lower limb amputation and identified 12 measures of global mental function, 1 measure of sensory function and pain, 1 measure of cardiovascular and respiratory function, and 2 measures of neuromuscular and movement function. Deathe and colleagues[4] reviewed measures of activity applicable to lower limb amputees and identified 4 walking tests, 1 mobility grading, 5 generic activity of daily living (ADL) and mobility measures, and 7 amputee-specific measures. Lindner and colleagues[5] reviewed outcome measures applicable for upper limb amputees, including 1 measure for subjects of all ages, 5 pediatric measures, and 2 adult measures. Most upper limb instruments measured activity and participation, while 2 measures also measured quality of life. These reviews all highlighted the lack of information about instrument responsiveness. **Table 1** summarizes the recommendations made by the authors of these reviews.

This article provides an update on the development of outcome instruments that are suitable for prosthetic practice, focusing on instruments published in English that are suitable for adult populations. The authors highlight recently published information about the psychometric properties of these instruments, especially responsiveness, and provide updated recommendations as to their suitability for clinical practice.

REVIEW METHODS

The authors replicated the search strategy described by Condie and colleagues[1] for publications from January 2006 to May 2013, and the search strategy described by Wright[2] from January 2009 to May 2013 using PubMed and CINAHL. Articles were included if they proposed a new outcome instrument or evaluated an existing outcome instrument, helping to provide insight into the instrument's performance. Articles were excluded if they were not about outcome instruments or an application of an instrument as part of a research study, were written in a language other than English, or were about an instrumented outcome measurement system. Also excluded were reports about validation of instruments translated into languages other than English.

SEARCH RESULTS

The search identified 36 articles that met the inclusion criteria spanning 37 unique instruments. An additional 13 relevant articles were identified by hand searching the references cited in these articles. These articles brought the number of unique instruments to 43. From this list, the authors identified articles in English with adult populations of prosthesis users that reported evidence of reliability, validity, and sensitivity to change. A mixture of amputation-specific instruments and those developed for general populations that measure constructs suitable for use by prosthetists was sought. **Table 2** summarizes the final list of 24 instruments reviewed in this article. The instrument summaries are organized by level of amputation (lower vs upper limb) and then by construct measured (mobility, function, quality of life, and patient satisfaction).

LOWER LIMB AMPUTATION–SPECIFIC FUNCTIONAL INSTRUMENTS
Prosthesis Evaluation Questionnaire—Mobility Scale (PEQ-MS and PEQ-MS 12/5)

The PEQ is an 82-item questionnaire comprising 9 scales, which was developed to assess function and prosthesis-related quality of life.[6] Miller and colleagues[7] subsequently combined the ambulation and transfer items of the PEQ to form a 13-item mobility scale, dubbed the PEQ-MS, and altered the response format from the original visual analog scale (VAS) to an 11-step rating scale. These investigators reported a Cronbach's α of 0.95 and good 4-week, test-retest reliability (intraclass correlation coefficient [ICC] = 0.77). The PEQ-MS also demonstrated convergent validity with the 2 Minute Walk Test (2MWT, r = 0.5), Timed Up and Go (TUG, r = 0.5), and Activities-Specific Balance Confidence (ABC) Scale (r = 0.82–0.85), and distinguished between different groups on clinically important variables including amputation etiology, walking distance, automatic walking, prosthetic wearing time, and mobility device use.

Franchignoni and colleagues[8] assessed the PEQ-MS rating categories, unidimensionality, construct validity, and reliability using Rasch analysis, administering the PEQ-MS by mail to 123 persons with transfemoral and transtibial amputation discharged from a national rehabilitation hospital. The instrument was revised from 13 to 12 items and the response categories collapsed from 11 to 5. The resulting PEQ-MS 12/5 has excellent person-separation reliability (0.95), excellent item-separation reliability (0.98), and good internal consistency (Cronbach's α = 0.96), results comparable with those of the original PEQ-MS. As reported by Franchignoni and colleagues[8] the PEQ-MS 12/5 correlated strongly with the Locomotor Capabilities Index (LCI) (r^2 = 0.78) and moderately with items from the Prosthetic Profile of the Amputee (PPA): frequency of prosthetic wear (r^2 = 0.59), prosthetic wear indoors and outdoors (r^2 = 0.41 and 0.43, respectively), and distance walked nonstop (r^2 = 0.48). Construct validity was supported by a logical hierarchy of item difficulty for both the PEQ-MS and the PEQ-MS 12/5.

Resnik and Borgia[9] recruited a convenience sample of 44 lower limb prosthesis users with transfemoral, knee disarticulation, and transtibial amputations, and administered the PEQ twice within 1 week. The average PEQ-MS score was 5.6 ± 0.9 (range: 3.5–7.0) on the first occasion and 5.4 ± 1.0 (range: 3.4–7.0) on the second occasion. PEQ-MS total ICC was 0.85 (95% confidence interval [CI] = 0.74–0.92), comparable with the previously reported value of 0.77.[7] Standard error of the mean (SEM) was 0.3 and minimal detectable change at the 90% CI (MDC90) was 0.8.

Hafner and colleagues[10] administered the PEQ-MS to 942 persons with lower limb loss (mean age 54 years, standard deviation [SD] = 14) with a mean PEQ-MS score of

Table 1
Published instrument summaries related to upper and lower limb prosthetics

Instrument	Lower Limb Prostheses			Upper Limb Prostheses		
	Condie et al,[1] 1996	Hebert et al,[3] 2009	Deathe et al,[4] 2009	Wright,[2] 2009	Lindner et al,[5] 2010	This Review
Lower Limb Mobility/Function						
Activity-Specific Balance Confidence Scale (ABC Scale)	—	R	—	—	—	N
Amputee Activity Score (AAS)	R	—	N	—	—	—
Amputee Body Image Scale (ABIS)	—	R	—	—	—	—
Amputee Mobility Predictor (AMPPRO)	R	—	N	—	—	R
Barthel Index	N	—	R (older dysvascular amputees only)	—	—	—
Berg Balance Scale (BBS)	—	—	—	—	—	N
Clinical Outcome Variables Scale (COVS)	—	—	N	—	—	—
Engagement in Everyday Activities Involving Revealing the Body (EEARB)	—	N	—	—	—	—
Functional Mobility Assessment (FMA)	R	—	—	—	—	—
Frenchay Activities Index (FAI)	N	—	—	—	—	—
Functional Independence Measure (FIM)	N	—	N	—	—	—
Houghton Scale	R	—	R	—	—	—
Locomotor Capabilities Index (LCI)	R (LCI & LCI-5)	—	R	—	—	N
Multidimensional Body-Self Relations Questionnaire (MBSRQ)	—	N	—	—	—	—
Office of Population Census and Survey Scale (OPCS)	N	—	—	—	—	—
Orthotics and Prosthetics Users' Survey Lower Extremity Functional Status (OPUS-LEFS)	—	—	—	—	—	N
Patient-Specific Functional Scale (PSFS)	—	—	—	—	—	R
Prosthetic Profile of the Amputee (PPA)	r	—	—	—	—	—

Questionnaire for Persons with a Transfemoral Amputation (Q-TFA)	—	—	N	—	—	—
Rivermead Mobility Index (RMI)	N	—	N	—	—	—
Russek's Code	N	—	—	—	—	—
Special Interest Group in Amputee Mobility (SIGAM)	R	—	R (classification measure only)	—	—	—
L Test of Functional Mobility (L Test)	—	—	R	—	—	R
Timed Up and Go (TUG)	R	—	R	—	—	R
10 Meter Walk Test (10mWT)	R	—	R	—	—	N
2 Minute Walk Test (2MWT)	R	—	R	—	—	R
6 Minute Walk Test (6MWT)	R	—	—	—	—	R
Wheelchair Skills Test (WST)	—	—	N	—	—	—
Quality of Life						
Amputation-Related Body Image Scale (ARBIS)	N	—	—	—	—	—
Attitudes to Artificial Limbs Questionnaire (AALQ)	N	N	—	—	—	—
Body Image Questionnaire (BIQ)	N	N	—	—	—	—
Patient Generated Index (PGI)	N	—	—	—	—	—
Short-Form Healthy Survey (SF36/SF12)	N	—	—	N	—	—
Sickness Impact Profile (SIP)	N	—	—	—	—	—
Orthotics and Prosthetics National Outcomes Tool (OPOT)	r	—	—	—	—	—
Orthotics and Prosthetics Users' Survey Health-Related Quality of Life (OPUS-HRQOL)	—	—	—	—	—	N
Orthotic and Prosthetic User's Survey Satisfaction with Device and Services	—	—	—	—	—	N
Prosthesis Evaluation Questionnaire (PEQ)	r	—	—	—	—	—
Prosthesis Evaluation Questionnaire Mobility Scale (PEQ-MS)	—	—	R	—	—	R

(continued on next page)

Table 1
(continued)

Instrument	Lower Limb Prostheses			Upper Limb Prostheses		
	Condie et al,[1] 1996	Hebert et al,[3] 2009	Deathe et al,[4] 2009	Wright,[2] 2009	Lindner et al,[5] 2010	This Review
Perceived Social Stigma Scale (PSSS)	N	—	—	—	—	—
Trinity Amputation and Prosthesis Experience Scales (TAPES)	N	—	—	R (a)	R	R
Adult Upper Limb Function						
Activities Measure for Upper Limb Amputees (AM-ULA)	—	—	—	—	—	R
Assessment of Capacity for Myoelectric Control (ACMC)	—	—	—	R (a,c)	R	N
Box and Block Test (BBT)	—	—	—	—	—	R
Disabilities of Arm, Shoulder, and Hand (DASH)	—	—	—	R (a)	—	R
Jebsen-Taylor Test of Hand Function (JTHF)	—	—	—	—	—	R
Nottingham Health Profile (NHP)	—	—	—	N	—	—
Orthotics and Prosthetics Users' Survey Upper Extremity Functional Status (OPUS-UEFS)	—	—	—	R (a)	R	N
Southampton Hand Assessment Profile (SHAP)	—	—	—	N	—	—
Pediatric Upper Limb Function						
ABILHAND-KIDS	—	—	—	R (c)	—	—
Assisting Hand Assessment (AHA)	—	—	—	R (c)	—	—
Child Amputee Prosthetic Project-Functional Status Inventory (CAPP-FSI)	—	—	N	N	N	N
Pediatric Quality of Life Inventory (PedsQL)	—	—	—	N	—	—

Pediatric Orthopedic Data Collection Outcomes Instrument (PODCI)	—	—	—	N
Prosthetic Upper Extremity Functional Index (PUFI)	—	—	R (c)	R
Unilateral Below Elbow Test (UBET)	—	—	N	N
University of New Brunswick (UNB) Test	—	—	R (c)	N
Global Mental Function: Depression or Emotional Status				
Beck Depression Inventory (BDI)	—	N	—	—
Center for Epidemiological Studies–Depression Scale (CES-D)	—	R	—	—
General Health Questionnaire (GHQ-28)	—	R	—	—
Geriatric Depression Survey (GDS)	—	N	—	—
Hospital Anxiety and Depression Scale (HADS)	—	N	—	—
Sensory Function and Pain				
Socket Comfort Score (SCS)	—	R	—	R
Cardiovascular and Respiratory				
One-leg cycling test (Vo$_{2max}$ Anaerobic Threshold)	r	—	—	—
Neuromusculoskeletal and Movement				
Walking speed (instrumented assessment)	r	—	—	—
Postural sway (instrumented assessment)	r	—	—	—

Abbreviations: a, adults; c, children; R, recommended for clinical practice; N, not recommended for use with amputees; r, recommended for research only.

Table 2
Summary of outcome instruments by outcome construct

Construct	Performance Measure	Patient-Reported Outcome	Lower Limb	Upper Limb	Norms Available Condition Specific	Norms Available General Population	Evidence of Responsiveness or Sensitivity
Activity							
10mWT	X	—	X	—	—	—	—
ABC Scale	—	X	X	—	—	—	—
AMPRO	X	—	X	—	16	—	SEM, MDC90[16]
ACMC	X	—	—	X	—	—	—
AM-ULA	X	—	—	X	—	—	MDC[32]
BBS	X	—	X	—	—	—	—
BBT	X	—	—	X	—	34	MDC90[33]
JTHF	X	—	—	X	—	—	MDC[33]
LCI	X	—	X	—	—	—	—
L-Test	X	—	X	—	—	—	SEM[17]
OPUS-LEFS	—	X	X	—	—	—	—
OPUS-UEFS	—	X	—	X	—	—	—
PSFS	—	X	X	—	—	—	SEM, MDC90[16]
PEQ-MS	—	X	X	—	9	—	SEM, MDC90[16]
PPA	—	X	X	—	—	—	—

PUFI	—	X	X	—	X	—
6MWT	X	—	X	—	X	SEM, MDC90[16]
TUG	X	—	X	—	X	SEM, MDC90[16]
TAPES-R	—	X	X	—	X	MDC[31]
2MWT	X	—	X	—	X	SEM, MDC90[16] Cutoffs 130–150 m[25]
Health-Related Quality of Life						
OPUS-HRQOL	—	X	X	—	X	—
PROMIS	—	X	—	—	—	See PROMIS Web site
SCS	—	X	X	—	X	Wilcoxon z = 74.16, P<.001[38]
Patient Satisfaction						
OPUS-Satisfaction	—	X	X	—	X	—

Abbreviations: 2MWT, 2 Minute Walk Test; 6MWT, 6 Minute Walk Test; 10mWT, 10 Meter Walk Test; ABC Scale, Activities-Specific Balance Confidence Scale; ACMC, Assessment of Capacity for Myoelectric Control; AMPRO, Amputee Mobility Predictor; AM-ULA, Activities Measure for Upper Limb Amputees; BBS, Berg Balance Scale; BBT, Box and Block Test; JTHF, Jebsen-Taylor Test of Hand Function; LCI, Locomotor Capabilities Index; L-Test, L-Test of Functional Mobility; MDC90, minimal detectable change at the 90% confidence interval; OPUS-HRQOL, Orthotics and Prosthetics Users' Survey Health-Related Quality of Life; OPUS-LEFS, Orthotics and Prosthetics Users' Survey Lower Extremity Functional Status; OPUS-UEFS, Orthotics and Prosthetics Users' Survey Upper Extremity Functional Status; PEQ-MS, Prosthesis Evaluation Questionnaire Mobility Scale; PPA, Prosthetic Profile of the Amputee; PROMIS, Patient-Reported Outcome Measurement Information System; PSFS, Patient-Specific Functional Scale; PUFI, Prosthetic Upper Extremity Functional Index; SCS, Socket Comfort Score; SEM, standard error of the mean; TAPES-R, Trinity Amputation and Prosthesis Experience Scales—Revised; TUG, Timed Up and Go.

33.2 (SD = 10.3). Mobility was related to etiology and level of amputation; 4 subgroups based on amputation level (transtibial/transfemoral) and etiology (trauma/dysvascular) differed significantly on PEQ-MS scores. Persons with dysvascular transfemoral amputations reported significantly worse mobility (mean = 26.3, SD = 11.1), whereas persons with traumatic transtibial amputation reported significantly better mobility (mean = 37.0, SD = 9.6).

Locomotor Capabilities Index (LCI, LCI-5, LCI10-4)

The LCI is a component of the PPA that has been independently validated[11,12] and used widely.[1] The LCI contains 14 items that assess locomotor skills and level of independence in using a lower limb prosthesis.[13] Each item is scored on a 4-point ordinal scale yielding a total maximum score of 42, with maximum subscores of 21 for basic and advanced locomotor skills. Higher scores indicate better locomotor abilities. The LCI-5 uses a 5-point rating scale to better report the use of walking aids.[14] Condie and colleagues[1] reported that both the LCI and LCI-5 demonstrated good internal consistency, test-retest reliability, and construct validity, with the LCI-5 reducing the LCI ceiling effect by 50%.

Franchignoni and colleagues[15] assessed the psychometric properties of the LCI-5 using Rasch analysis; they administered the LCI-5 by mailed survey to 123 persons with transfemoral and transtibial amputation discharged from a national rehabilitation hospital, and reduced the rating scale to 4. The revised LCI10-4 demonstrated excellent person-separation reliability (0.94) and excellent item-separation reliability (0.98), results comparable with those of the LCI-5. As reported by Franchignoni and colleagues,[15] the LCI-5 correlated strongly with the PEQ-MS ($r^2 = 0.77$) and moderately with the PPA items prosthetic wear ($r^2 = 0.47$), prosthetic wear indoors and outdoors ($r^2 = 0.34$ and 0.42, respectively), and distance walked nonstop ($r^2 = 0.51$). Construct validity was supported by a logical hierarchy of item difficulty for both the LCI-5 and LCI10-4.

Amputee Mobility Predictor (AMP, AMPPRO, and AMPnoPro)

The AMP measures ambulatory potential of people with lower limb amputations with (AMPPRO) and without a prosthesis (AMPnoPro); published psychometric studies are available only for the AMPPRO.[16] The AMP consists of 21 items that evaluate transfers, sitting and standing balance, and gait skills. It demonstrates good interrater and intrarater reliability,[16] and concurrent validity has been established with the 6 Minute Walk Test (6MWT) and Amputee Activity Survey (AAS).[16] The AMPPRO predicts distance walked in 6 minutes[16] and distinguishes Medicare Functional Classification Levels (k-levels),[16] although wide score distributions preclude cutoff scores.[4]

Resnik and Borgia[9] recruited a convenience sample of 44 lower limb prosthesis users with transfemoral, knee disarticulation, and transtibial amputations, and administered the AMPPRO twice within 1 week. The average AMPPRO score was 40 ± 4 (range: 28–45) on the first occasion and 41 ± 4 (range: 29–46) on the second occasion. AMPPRO total ICC was 0.88 (95% CI = 0.79–0.93), comparable with previous reports of 0.96 to 0.98.[16] SEM was 1.5 and MDC90 was 3.4.

L-Test of Functional Mobility (L-Test)

The L-Test is an adaptation of the TUG, intended to assess basic mobility skills in individuals with unilateral lower limb amputation. It was designed to reduce the ceiling effect of the TUG observed in younger, fitter elderly amputees.[17] It incorporates 2 transfers and 4 turns, of which at least one is to the opposite side with a total distance covered of 20 m. The score is the time taken to stand from an armless chair, walk 10 m in the shape of an L at usual walking speed, turn 180°, and return 10 m in the shape of an L to a seated position. Amount and type of encouragement is standardized. In 93 unilateral transtibial and transfemoral amputees, interrater reliability (ICC) was 0.96 (95% CI = 0.94–0.97) and intrarater reliability was 0.97 (95% CI = 0.93–0.97).[17] The interrater SEM was 3.0 seconds.[17] Concurrent validity is supported with the TUG (r = 0.93), 10 Meter Walk Test (10mWT; r = 0.97), 2MWT (r = −0.86), ABC Scale (r = −0.48), Frenchay Activities Index (FAI; r = −0.54), and PEQ-MS (r = −0.22).[17] The L-Test discriminates between clinically meaningful groups, with higher mean times observed for persons who are older (>55 years = 39.7 ± 17.1 seconds; <55 years = 25.4 ± 6.8 seconds), do not use a walking aid (unaided = 43.3 ± 17.5 seconds; walking aid = 25.5 ± 6.4 seconds), have vascular amputations (vascular = 42.0 ± 17.8 seconds; traumatic = 26.4 ± 7.8 seconds), and transfemoral amputations (transfemoral = 41.7 ± 16.8 seconds; transtibial = 29.5 ± 12.8 seconds).[17]

Orthotics and Prosthetics Users' Survey Lower Extremity Functional Status (OPUS-LEFS)

The LEFS contained in the OPUS was developed with clinician and patient input and a comprehensive literature search of generic, orthotic-specific, and prosthetic-specific outcome instruments. Selecting items from a variety of existing instruments, Heinemann and colleagues[18] proposed a set of 20 items rated on a 5-point rating scale. OPUS items were evaluated with a telephone field test of past recipients of orthotic and prosthetic services with a combined sample of 164 subjects, including 80 adults and 84 children. Rasch analysis was used to evaluate internal consistency and content validity.[18] The easiest items are "get on and off toilet," "get up from a chair," and "walk indoors." Items of average difficulty include "pick up an object from the floor while standing," "get on and off an escalator," and "walk outdoors on uneven ground." The most difficult items are "walk up to 2 hours" and "run one block." The items were well targeted to the sample. Internal consistency was excellent (0.94 person-separation reliability; 0.98 item-separation reliability).

Jarl and colleagues[19] added 7 items to the LEFS: jog one-half hour, jog 1 hour, participate in vigorous sports for 1 hour, participate in vigorous sports for one-half hour, stand and walk for half a working day, go shopping for half a day, and stand up for 1 hour; deleted 1 item; and collapsed the rating scale options to 4 levels (cannot perform, difficult, easy, very easy). In a sample of 282 prosthesis and orthosis users, they reported excellent internal consistency (Cronbach's α = 0.96) and minimal ceiling and floor effects. There was only slight evidence for gender-related and age-related differential item functioning.

GENERIC LOWER LIMB FUNCTIONAL INSTRUMENTS
Timed Up and Go (TUG)

The TUG test is a performance measure of mobility and balance. Participants start seated with their backs against the chair and their arms resting on the chair arms. On the word "go," the participant stands, walks 3 m at a normal pace, turns, walks back to the chair, and sits down. Participants may use their standard walking aid. Time is measured in seconds. Shorter time to complete the task indicates better ability. Administration time is less than 5 minutes. Equipment includes a standard armchair (seat height 46 cm; arm height 67 cm) and a stopwatch.

The TUG has demonstrated good intrarater (r = 0.93) and interrater (r = 0.96) reliability, and evidence of validity for a sample of 46 patients age 60 years or older with unilateral transtibial or transfemoral amputation because of peripheral vascular disease.[20] ICC was estimated to be 0.88 (95% CI = 0.80–0.94), the SEM was estimated at 1.6 and the MDC90 at 3.6.[9] Convergent validity was demonstrated with the Houghton Scale ($r = -0.60$), the PEQ-MS ($r = -0.50$), and the LCI ($r = -0.64$).[7]

Berg Balance Scale (BBS)

The BBS is a 14-item performance measure of static sitting and standing balance, and fall risk in adult populations. The 14 tasks include sitting, standing, reaching, leaning over, turning and looking over each shoulder, turning in a complete circle, and stepping. Items are scored on a rating scale of 0 to 4 with a total score range of 0 to 56. Total scores of 0 to 20 indicate a high risk for falls, 21 to 40 indicate a moderate risk, and 41 to 56 indicate a low risk in adults with vestibular dysfunction.[21] Administration time is 15 to 20 minutes. Required equipment includes a stopwatch, chair with armrests, measuring tape/ruler, object to pick up off the floor, and step stool.

Interrater reliability is reported as ICC = 0.94 and internal consistency as Cronbach's α = 0.83 in a sample of 30 persons with unilateral transtibial (n = 13), unilateral transfemoral (n = 14), or bilateral (n = 3) lower limb amputation of dysvascular (n = 7), traumatic (n = 14), infectious (n = 6), or congenital (n = 3) origin.[22] A minor ceiling effect was noted. High convergent validity was demonstrated with the ABC Scale ($r = 0.63$), PEQ-MS ($r = 0.58$), 2MWT ($r = 0.68$), and L-Test ($r = -0.80$), all statistically significant at $P<.001$.[22]

Activities-Specific Balance Confidence Scale (ABC Scale)

The ABC Scale is a 16-item self-report measure of confidence in performing various ADLs without falling. Items are scored on a rating scale from 0 to 100, with higher scores reflecting higher levels of balance confidence. An average score is calculated by summing all item scores and dividing by the total number of items. Administration time is 10 to 20 minutes. The ABC Scale is recommended by Hebert and colleagues[3] for use in clinical practice because it provides useful clinical information despite limited evidence of its validity.

The 4-week test-retest reliability of the average score was estimated with an ICC of 0.91 (95% CI = 0.84–0.95) in a sample of 50 persons with transtibial (n = 38) and transfemoral (n = 12) amputations.[23] Convergent validity was demonstrated with a positive association ($r = 0.72$, 95% CI = 0.56–0.84) with the 2MWT and a negative association ($r = -0.70$, 95% CI = -0.82 to -0.53) with the TUG.[23]

A 5-point rating scale was found to be more appropriate for a sample of 448 community-living adults 50 years or older with unilateral lower limb amputation, whereby the Cronbach's α was 0.94 and the SEM ranged from 0.27 to 0.40.[24]

Patient-Specific Functional Scale (PSFS)

The PSFS requires respondents to list up to 5 major activities that they find difficult to perform because of conditions and disabilities, including amputation. Thereafter, respondents rate their ability to complete the activities using a 10-point rating scale whereby 0 is "can't perform at all" and 10 is "can perform fully." The mean response is the PSFS summary score. In a sample of 44 patients with unilateral lower limb amputation, the ICC for the summary score was 0.83 (95% CI = 0.71–0.90), SEM was 4.8, and MDC90 was 11.2.[9] Floor and ceiling effects were minimal.

Timed Walking Tests (2MWT, 6MWT)

Timed walking tests measure endurance over a set period. Participants walk along a long straight corridor for 2 or 6 minutes at a self-selected walking speed. Participants may use a mobility aid and rest if needed. Shorter walking tests are more suitable for patients with severe disabilities. The only required equipment is a stopwatch.

In a sample of 44 patients with unilateral lower limb amputation, the 2MWT ICC was estimated at 0.83 (95% CI = 0.71–0.90), SEM was 48.5, and MDC90 was 112.5.[9] In another sample of 64 patients with unilateral lower limb amputation it was reported that the 2MWT was the best predictor of prosthetic walking limitations in comparison with the BBS, Functional Reach test, one-leg balance on the unaffected limb, Tandem test, TUG, and Modified Houghton Scale. No floor or ceiling effects were seen in this sample.[25]

In a sample of 44 patients with unilateral lower limb amputation, the 6MWT ICC was estimated at 0.97 (95% CI = 0.95–0.99), SEM was 63.6, and MDC90 was 147.5.[9] Evidence of validity includes slower walking speeds by transfemoral versus transtibial groups.[26]

Distance Walking Tests (10mWT)

The 10mWT assesses walking speed in meters per second at a usual pace from a standing start. Required equipment includes a stopwatch and a clear pathway of at least 14 m. In a sample of 93 individuals with unilateral amputation (74% transtibial, 26% transfemoral) the 10mWT was highly correlated with the L-Test (r = 0.97).[17]

UPPER LIMB AMPUTATION–SPECIFIC FUNCTIONAL INSTRUMENTS
Assessment of Capacity for Myoelectric Control (ACMC)

The ACMC is an observational rating of performance of 30 bimanual movements during a self-chosen ADL for users of myoelectric prosthetic hands. Items include gripping, holding, releasing, and coordinating objects between hands. Scoring reflects quality of movement control along a 4-point scale ranging from "not capable" to "spontaneously capable."[27] Rasch analysis of a sample of 96 children and adults aged 2 to 57 years (mean age 11 years) suggests the ACMC is sufficiently unidimensional[27,28] and is an internally consistent measure (person reliability = 0.97).[28] The ACMC discriminates a wide range of ability levels (person-separation index 5.21, item-separation index 7.28),[28] and is well targeted to respondents (mean person ability 0.48 logits, SD = 2.81 logits).[28]

Interrater and intrarater reliability were evaluated in a study with three occupational therapists and a sample of 26 persons 2 to 40 years old with upper limb amputation. Two raters were students with either no previous experience or 10 weeks of experience, and 1 was a clinician with 15 years of experience with myoelectric training. Intrarater reliability was related to level of experience: raters with more experience had excellent agreement (mean κ = 0.81), whereas the novice clinician had only good agreement (mean κ = 0.60).[29] Interrater reliability was higher between the 2 most experienced clinicians (κ = 0.60) than between the 2 raters with the least experience (κ = 0.47).[29] This study demonstrates the importance of training and practice of evaluations in administering this instrument reliably. Raters must complete training to access the ACMC scoring Web site.

Orthotics and Prosthetics Users' Survey Upper Extremity Functional Status (OPUS-UEFS)

The UEFS contained in the OPUS[18] is a patient-reported measure of upper limb functional status. The original UEFS was composed of 14 bilateral and 9 unilateral activities. Examples include drinking from a paper cup, buttoning a shirt, and tying shoelaces. The 5-point rating scale ranges from "cannot perform" to "very easy."

Burger and colleagues[30] completed the first validation study with a convenience sample of 61 adult upper limb amputees, 4 of whom did not have a prosthesis. Rasch analysis of the UEFS identified 2 misfitting items and 2 items with high residual correlations. The resulting 19-item UEFS 2.0 demonstrated excellent reliability with item-separation reliability of 0.96 and person-separation reliability of 0.88. The UEFS 2.0 is mistargeted on its intended population, prompting the developers to recommend development of additional items of greater difficulty.[30]

Jarl and colleagues[19] evaluated 6 additional items in a sample of 134 users of upper limb orthoses and prostheses. The new items included taking bank notes from a wallet, twisting a lid off a small bottle, and sharpening a pencil. One original item misfit and one new item demonstrated a high residual correlation. The resulting 27-item scale showed excellent reliability for orthosis users, but the responses from prosthesis users (n = 54) were excluded because of inconsistent response patterns, perhaps because of confusion about using a prosthesis during one-handed tasks. The investigators recommend clarifying the instructions in future validation studies.[19]

Resnik and Borgia[31] evaluated a revised version of the UEFS with a sample of 73 adults with unilateral and bilateral upper limb amputations. This version contained 22 of the original items; it demonstrated good test-retest reliability of the overall person-level summary score (ICC 5 0.80, 95% CI 5 0.68–0.87), but moderate test-retest reliability of the UEFS use scores (ICC 5 0.65, 95% CI 5 0.47–0.77). It did not distinguish performance by level of amputation, perhaps because respondents may answer items with or without prosthesis use, and because many items can be completed using the unimpaired arm. The investigators recommended modifying items to ask specifically how easily a task can be completed with and without the prosthesis.[31]

Activities Measure for Upper Limb Amputees (AM-ULA)

The AM-ULA is an 18-item, clinician-rated assessment of multistep, functional tasks. Items assess removing a T-shirt, tying shoelaces, using a fork, and folding a bath towel. Clinicians rate 5 aspects of performance for each task including the extent of completion, speed of completion, quality of movement, skillfulness and control of the prosthesis, and independence, using a scale of 0 to 4 points that ranges from "unable" to "excellent." The lowest category score serves as the overall item score. A detailed protocol for administration is available and is recommended by the instrument developers.[32]

In a cohort study of 49 adults with upper limb amputation using any type of prosthesis, Resnik and colleagues[32] reported that the AM-ULA demonstrates good test-retest reliability (ICC = 0.88–0.91) and interrater reliability (ICC = 0.84–0.89). It demonstrated acceptable internal consistency, with Cronbach's α ranging from 0.89 to 0.91. Moderate convergent validity (r = 0.63) was established with the Box and Blocks Test (BBT). Evidence of known-groups validity is provided by significant differences in scores across level of amputation. MDC was estimated at 3.7 points with a 90% CI and 4.4 points with a 95% CI. Norms have not been established.

Box and Blocks Test (BBT)

The BBT is a quick assessment of unilateral manual dexterity.[31] Standardized testing materials, administration procedures, and prefabricated test sets can be purchased.[33] Equipment includes an open box with a center partition, 150 wooden blocks, and a stopwatch. The score is the number of blocks the participant is able to pick up, transport over the partition, and release within 60 seconds. Normative data are available for able-bodied adults older than 20 and children from 6 to 19 years old.[33] The BBT demonstrated excellent test-retest reliability in a sample of 73 adults with upper limb amputation (ICC = 0.91, 95% CI = 0.85–0.95) and known group validity by amputation level.[31] MDC90 for upper limb amputees is 6.49 and MDC95 is 7.77. Floor and ceiling effects were not observed. Although interrater reliability has been established for raters of subjects from the general population (r = 0.99 for left-hand testing and r = 1.00 for right-hand testing),[33] testing has not been completed for raters of subjects using an upper limb prosthesis. Convergent validity with amputee-specific instruments has not been demonstrated.

Jebsen-Taylor Test of Hand Function (JTHF)

The JTHF is a generic dexterity test that has been validated for use with upper limb amputees.[31] Similarly to the BBT, standardized materials are needed to complete the tests, and the test kit can be made by following instructions found in the original article[34] or purchased. The JTHF comprises 7 subtests, including writing, card turning, picking up and placing small objects, stacking, simulated feeding, and moving large, light, and heavy objects. Resnik and colleagues[31] modified the scoring so that the time to complete each subtest was capped at 2 minutes and items completed per second were scored. Using a convenience sample of 73 adults with upper limb amputation, Resnik and colleagues[31] reported that test-retest reliability of subtests ranged from acceptable to excellent (ICC = 0.53–0.92), and MDCs ranged from 0.09 to 0.18 items per second with a 90% CI and 0.10 to 0.21 items per second at a 95% CI. Known group validity for amputation levels was statistically significant. The investigators reported floor and ceiling effects for 3 subtests.[31]

LOWER LIMB AMPUTATION–SPECIFIC HEALTH-RELATED QUALITY OF LIFE
Socket Comfort Score (SCS)

Poor socket comfort is possibly the most common issue experienced by prosthesis users. Like pain, comfort is subjective and difficult to measure. Therefore, it may be appropriate to adapt pain-measurement methods such as the numerical rating scale (NRS)[35,36] for quantifying and communicating socket-fit comfort. Hanspal and colleagues[37] proposed a version of the NRS, called the SCS, which asks the standard question, "On a 0 to 10 scale, if 0 represents the most uncomfortable socket fit you can imagine, and 10 represents the most comfortable socket fit, how would you score the comfort of the socket fit of your artificial limb at the moment?" These investigators reported interrater reliability, criterion-related validity, sensitivity to change, and utility in clinical practice in 44 consecutive lower limb amputees.[37] The treating prosthetist collected SCS responses 3 times during the course of a single day, as did an independent prosthetist and a physician. Their ratings were highly correlated (Kendall τ 0.97–0.98, $P<.001$).[37] SCS responses were significantly correlated with assessments of socket fit by the treating prosthetist and with residual limb health by a physician (Kendall τ 0.51 and 0.48, $P<.001$).[37] There was sensitivity to change, with 76% (n = 22) of adjusted sockets demonstrating a significant improvement in the SCS of 1 to 5 points (Wilcoxon z = 74.16, $P<.001$).[37] The SCS is a simple, easy-to-administer measure that allows clinicians to quantify change in socket fit rather than relying on descriptive terms.

Trinity Amputation and Prosthesis Experience Scales—Revised (TAPES-R)

The TAPES-R is a 64-item, patient-reported measure of 3 aspects of psychosocial adjustment: (1) general adjustment, (2) social adjustment, and (3) adjustment to limitation and activity restrictions; and 2 aspects of satisfaction: (1) aesthetic and (2) functional satisfaction.[38] Administration typically requires no more than 15 minutes. Rating scales vary across subscale and reflect extent of agreement (strongly disagree, disagree, agree, strongly agree for adjustment items), extent of restriction (limited a lot, limited a little, not limited at all for activities), and level of satisfaction (dissatisfied, satisfied, very satisfied). Items within each subscale are summed and then averaged. The developers used confirmatory factor and Rasch analysis to identify and delete misfitting items and to select a simpler scoring algorithm. Internal consistency is good for general adjustment (0.82 person-separation reliability), social adjustment (0.79), adjustment to limitation (0.80) and activity restriction (0.86), and marginal for satisfaction with prosthesis subscales (0.72, 0.77). The developers reported small floor and ceiling effects in a community sample of 498 adult prosthesis users with primary etiology of peripheral vascular disease, traumatic injury, and cancer. Test-retest reliability has not been reported. Further research is required to develop norms. Resnik and Borgia[31] reported ICC = 0.86 (95% CI = 0.76–0.92) for the satisfaction scale over 1 week and MDC of 0.79 (90% CI) and 0.83 (95% CI).

Orthotics and Prosthetics Users' Survey Health-Related Quality of Life (OPUS-HRQOL)

The HRQOL module of the OPUS was developed concurrently with the other OPUS modules using a combined sample of 164 subjects, including 80 adults and 84 children.[18] It comprises 23 items that are evaluated with a 5-point rating scale ranging from "all of the time" to "none of the time." Rating-scale analysis of the items supports the construct validity of the items. The easiest items to endorse are "how often during the past week have you been happy?"; "how often during the past week have you felt calm and peaceful?" and "how often during the past week did you have a lot of energy?" Items of average difficulty include "how often during the past week have you felt downhearted and depressed?"; "how much does pain interfere with your activities (including both work outside the home and household duties)?"; and "how much does your physical condition restrict your ability to do chores?" The most difficult items are "how often during the past week did you feel worn out?" and "how often during the past week did you feel tired?" The items are reasonably targeted to the sample, and demonstrated good internal consistency, with person-separation reliability (similar to Cronbach's α) of 0.88.

Jarl and colleagues[19] administered the HRQOL items to a sample of 275 prosthesis and orthosis users. Based on a principal-component analysis, they decided to split the items into a 6-item Restrictions and a 10-item Emotions subscales because of item misfit. Internal consistency was very good for both subscales (person reliability = 0.89 for both subscales, item reliability = 0.97 for the Restrictions subscale and 0.99 for the Emotions subscale). There was no floor effect, although 10.3% of the sample was at the ceiling of the Restrictions subscale and 2.5% were at the ceiling of the Emotions subscale.

GENERIC HEALTH-RELATED QUALITY OF LIFE INSTRUMENTS

Sinha and Van Den Heuvel[39] reviewed quality of life (QOL) in lower limb amputees and described 26 studies that used 12 QOL measures, including the SF36, RAND36, Nottingham Health Profile, Sickness Impact Profile, WHOQOLBref, EuroQuol, PEQ, VAS, and QOL ladder. In the interests of brevity, descriptions are provided here of generic and amputation-specific QOL instruments not reviewed previously.

Patient-Reported Outcomes Measurement Information System (PROMIS)

The National Institutes of Health (NIH), as part of its Roadmap for Medical Research, funded the development of PROMIS.[40] This initiative developed generic measures of patient-reported outcomes in physical, emotional, and social functioning domains. Rehabilitation stakeholders, including patients with limb loss, were engaged actively in its development.[41] Constructs relevant to prosthetic practice include pain, fatigue, depression, anxiety, sleep disruption, pain interference, and positive and negative illness impact, among others. The developers used Item Response Theory to develop and improve the item banks. The item banks can be administered using computer adaptive testing (CAT) through the NIH Assessment Center, or as short forms, without loss of scale precision or content validity. PROMIS methods of item bank development inspired development of the Prosthetic Limb Users Survey-Mobility (PLUS-M), and its development has included the assessment of domains of PROMIS for lower limb prosthesis users.[42]

The results from the PROMIS CATs are rescaled so that the average of the United States general population is 50 and its SD is 10. Thus, a person who has a PROMIS score of 40 is 1 SD below the United States average. For negatively worded concepts such as fatigue, a T-score of 60 is 1 SD worse than average (more fatigue) and a score of 40 is 1 SD better than average (less fatigue). For positively worded concepts such as positive psychosocial illness impact, a score of 60 is 1 SD better than average. PROMIS domains are assessed over the past 7 days. Additional psychometric information about PROMIS and ways to administer items is available at http://nihpromis. org/measures/domainframework.

AMPUTATION-SPECIFIC HEALTH-RELATED QUALITY OF LIFE INSTRUMENTS

Gallagher and Desmond[43] provide an excellent summary of considerations in selecting condition-specific quality of life instruments, which are not repeated here in the interests of brevity.

AMPUTATION-SPECIFIC PATIENT SATISFACTION INSTRUMENTS
Orthotics and Prosthetics Users' Survey Satisfaction with Device and Services

Two components of OPUS measure patient satisfaction: Satisfaction with Device and Satisfaction with Services.[18] The same sample used to develop the HRQOL, LEFS, and UEFS modules was also used for the patient satisfaction modules. For the Satisfaction with Device item set, the easiest items to endorse are "the weight of my prosthesis (or orthosis) is manageable" and "my prosthesis (or orthosis) is durable." Items of average difficulty were "it is easy to put on my prosthesis (or orthosis)" and "my clothes are free of wear and tear from my prosthesis (or orthosis)." The most difficult items to endorse are "my skin is free of abrasions and irritations" and "my prosthesis (or orthosis) is pain free to wear." The module has a positive skew and a pronounced ceiling effect, revealing that most patients are highly satisfied with their prosthesis.

Calibration of the Satisfaction with Services responses also yields acceptable measurement statistics. The items easiest to endorse are "I was shown the proper level of courtesy and respect by the staff" and "I received an appointment with a prosthetist/ orthotist within a reasonable amount of time." Items of average difficulty are "I am satisfied with the training I received in the use and maintenance of my prosthesis/ orthosis" and "the prosthetist/orthotist gave me the opportunity to express my concerns regarding my equipment." The items most difficult to endorse are "I was a partner in decision-making with clinic staff regarding my care and equipment" and "the prosthetist (orthotist) discussed problems I might encounter with my equipment." None of the items misfit the construct. As is common with many other satisfaction instruments, the items are mistargeted to the sample (mean measure of 2.91 logits), revealing a high level of satisfaction with services.

CONTROVERSIES AND FUTURE CONSIDERATIONS

For an outcome instrument to be clinically useful, the magnitude of score change be-tween repeated assessments should be able to reflect a real change in patients' clin-ical status. Few of the identified outcome instruments clearly state this magnitude. Further research on this issue is needed, as this will help the clinician to evaluate any improvement after intervention and to plan further treatment goals.

SUMMARY

Accreditors expect prosthetists to monitor patient outcomes as part of routine clinical practice, although they typically are satisfied with assessment of patient satisfaction. Outcomes of patient care can be rated by prosthetists when performance of tasks is important, or reported by patients when improving patient-centered care is important. Only a few instruments have been the subject of intensive psychometric development for amputee populations. Considerable work is still required to develop norms and define MDCs. Routine monitoring of outcomes allows clinicians to address patient concerns in a timely manner and to implement quality-improvement initiatives while fulfilling accreditation requirements.

ACKNOWLEDGMENTS

The authors thank Kyle Swensen for assistance with literature searches and Neal Michalik for assistance with preparation of the article.

REFERENCES

1. Condie E, Jones D, Treweek S, et al. A one-year national survey of patients having a lower limb amputation. Physiotherapy 1996;82(1):14–20.
2. Wright V. Prosthetic outcome measures for use with upper limb amputees: a sys-tematic review of the peer-reviewed literature, 1970 to 2009. J Prosthet Orthot 2009;21(9):P3–63.
3. Hebert JS, Wolfe DL, Miller WC, et al. Outcome measures in amputation rehabil-itation: ICF body functions. Disabil Rehabil 2009;31(19):1541–54.
4. Deathe AB, Wolfe DL, Devlin M, et al. Selection of outcome measures in lower extremity amputation rehabilitation: ICF activities. Disabil Rehabil 2009;31(18):1455–73.
5. Lindner HY, Natterlund BS, Hermansson LM. Upper limb prosthetic outcome measures: review and content comparison based on international classifica-tion of functioning, disability and health. Prosthet Orthot Int 2010;34(2):109–28.
6. Legro MW, Reiber GD, Smith DG, et al. Prosthesis evaluation questionnaire for persons with lower limb amputations: assessing prosthesis-related quality of life. Arch Phys Med Rehabil 1998;79(8):931–8.
7. Miller WC, Deathe AB, Speechley M. Lower extremity prosthetic mobility: a comparison of 3 self-report scales. Arch Phys Med Rehabil 2001;82(10):1432–40.
8. Franchignoni F, Giordano A, Ferriero G, et al. Measuring mobility in people with lower limb amputation: Rasch analysis of the mobility section of the prosthesis evaluation questionnaire. J Rehabil Med 2007;39(2):138–44.
9. Resnik L, Borgia M. Reliability of outcome measures for people with lower-limb amputations: distinguishing true change from statistical error. Phys Ther 2011;91(4):555–65.

10. Hafner B, Amtmann D, Abrahamson D, et al. Normative PEQ-MS and ABC scores among persons with lower limb loss. Paper presented at American Academy of Orthotists & Prosthetists 39th Annual Meeting and Scientific Symposium. Orlando (FL), February 20–23, 2013.

11. Gauthier-Gagnon C, Grise M, Lepage Y. The Locomotor capabilities index: content validity. Journal Rehabilitation Outcomes Measurement 1998;2(4):40–6.

12. Gauthier-Gagnon C, Grise MC. Prosthetic profile of the amputee questionnaire: validity and reliability. Arch Phys Med Rehabil 1994;75(12):1309–14.

13. Gauthier-Gagnon C, Grisé MC. Tools to measure outcome of people with a lower limb amputation: update on the PPA and LCI. J Prosthet Orthot 2006;18(6):P61–7.

14. Franchignoni F, Orlandini D, Ferriero G, et al. Reliability, validity, and responsiveness of the locomotor capabilities index in adults with lower-limb amputation undergoing prosthetic training. Arch Phys Med Rehabil 2004;85(5):743–8.

15. Franchignoni F, Giordano A, Ferriero G, et al. Rasch analysis of the Locomotor Capabilities Index-5 in people with lower limb amputation. Prosthet Orthot Int 2007;31(4):394–404.

16. Gailey RS, Roach KE, Applegate EB, et al. The amputee mobility predictor: an instrument to assess determinants of the lower-limb amputee's ability to ambulate. Arch Phys Med Rehabil 2002;83(5):613–27.

17. Deathe AB, Miller WC. The L test of functional mobility: measurement properties of a modified version of the timed "up & go" test designed for people with lower-limb amputations. Phys Ther 2005;85(7):626–35.

18. Heinemann AW, Bode RK, O'Reilly C. Development and measurement properties of the Orthotics and Prosthetics Users' Survey (OPUS): a comprehensive set of clinical outcome instruments. Prosthet Orthot Int 2003;27(3):191–206.

19. Jarl GM, Heinemann AW, Norling Hermansson LM. Validity evidence for a modified version of the orthotics and prosthetics users' survey. Disabil Rehabil Assist Technol 2012;7(6):469–78.

20. Schoppen T, Boonstra A, Groothoff JW, et al. The timed "up and go" test: reliability and validity in persons with unilateral lower limb amputation. Arch Phys Med Rehabil 1999;80(7):825–8.

21. Badke MB, Shea TA, Miedaner JA, et al. Outcomes after rehabilitation for adults with balance dysfunction. Arch Phys Med Rehabil 2004;85(2):227–33.

22. Major MJ, Fatone S, Roth EJ. Validity and reliability of the Berg Balance Scale for community-dwelling persons with lower limb amputation. Arch Phys Med Rehabil 2013. [Epub ahead of print].

23. Miller WC, Deathe AB, Speechley M. Psychometric properties of the Activities-specific Balance Confidence Scale among individuals with a lower-limb amputation. Arch Phys Med Rehabil 2003;84(5):656–61.

24. Sakakibara BM, Miller WC, Backman CL. Rasch analyses of the Activities-specific Balance Confidence Scale with individuals 50 years and older with lower-limb amputations. Arch Phys Med Rehabil 2011;92(8):1257–63.

25. Gremeaux V, Damak S, Troisgros O, et al. Selecting a test for the clinical assessment of balance and walking capacity at the definitive fitting state after unilateral amputation: a comparative study. Prosthet Orthot Int 2012;36(4):415–22.

26. Kark L, McIntosh AS, Simmons A. The use of the 6-min walk test as a proxy for the assessment of energy expenditure during gait in individuals with lower-limb amputation. Int J Rehabil Res 2011;34(3):227–34.

27. Hermansson LM, Fisher AG, Bernspang B, et al. Accoocment of capacity for myoelectric control: a new Rasch-built measure of prosthetic hand control. J Rehabil Med 2005;37(3):166–71.

28. Lindner HY, Linacre JM, Norling Hermansson LM. Assessment of capacity for myoelectric control: evaluation of construct and rating scale. J Rehabil Med 2009;41(6):467–74.
29. Hermansson LM, Bodin L, Eliasson AC. Intra- and inter-rater reliability of the assessment of capacity for myoelectric control. J Rehabil Med 2006;38(2):118–23.
30. Burger H, Franchignoni F, Heinemann AW, et al. Validation of the orthotics and prosthetics user survey upper extremity functional status module in people with unilateral upper limb amputation. J Rehabil Med 2008;40(5):393–9.
31. Resnik L, Borgia M. Reliability and validity of outcome measures for upper limb amputation. J Prosthet Orthot 2012;24(4):192–201.
32. Resnik L, Adams L, Borgia M, et al. Development and evaluation of the activities measure for upper limb amputees. Arch Phys Med Rehabil 2013;94(3):488–94.e4.
33. Mathiowetz V, Volland G, Kashman N, et al. Adult norms for the box and block test of manual dexterity. Am J Occup Ther 1985;39(6):386–91.
34. Jebsen RH, Taylor N, Trieschmann RB, et al. An objective and standardized test of hand function. Arch Phys Med Rehabil 1969;50(6):311–9.
35. Downie WW, Leatham PA, Rhind VM, et al. Studies with pain rating scales. Ann Rheum Dis 1978;37(4):378–81.
36. Karoly P, Jensen MP. Multimethod assessment of chronic pain. 1st edition. Oxford (NY): Pergamon Press; 1987.
37. Hanspal RS, Fisher K, Nieveen R. Prosthetic socket fit comfort score. Disabil Rehabil 2003;25(22):1278–80.
38. Gallagher P, Franchignoni F, Giordano A, et al. Trinity amputation and prosthesis experience scales: a psychometric assessment using classical test theory and Rasch analysis. Am J Phys Med Rehabil 2010;89(6):487–96.
39. Sinha R, Van Den Heuvel WJ. A systematic literature review of quality of life in lower limb amputees. Disabil Rehabil 2011;33(11):883–99.
40. Cella D, Riley W, Stone A, et al. The patient-reported outcomes measurement information system (PROMIS) developed and tested its first wave of adult self-reported health outcome item banks: 2005–2008. J Clin Epidemiol 2010;63(11): 1179–94.
41. Amtmann D, Cook KF, Johnson KL, et al. The PROMIS initiative: involvement of rehabilitation stakeholders in development and examples of applications in rehabilitation research. Arch Phys Med Rehabil 2011;92(Suppl 10):S12–9.
42. Hafner B, Amtmann D, Morgan S, et al. Health profiles of persons with lower limb loss. Paper presented at the International Society for Prosthetics and Orthotics World Congress. Hyderabad (India), February 4–7, 2013.
43. Gallagher P, Desmond D. Measuring quality of life in prosthetic practice: benefits and challenges. Prosthet Orthot Int 2007;31(2):167–76.

Ideal Functional Outcomes for Amputation Levels

Robert H. Meier III, MD[a],*, Danielle Melton, MD[b,c,d]

KEYWORDS

- Functional outcomes • Amputations • Classifications • Ideal

KEY POINTS

- Levels of amputations: To define amputation levels and how this relates to functional outcomes.
- The role of the rehabilitation team: Individual roles of the team members in accomplishing the rehabilitation of the amputee patient.
- Prosthetic candidacy: Based on comorbidities, compliance, energy expenditure, K-levels, and objective measures and subjective assessments.
- Therapy (physical, occupational, psychological, vocational): How each discipline contributes to the rehabilitation process.
- Ideal outcomes: Determining expected functional independence after an amputation.

LEVELS OF AMPUTATION

For both upper and lower limbs, amputations are classified into specific levels (**Fig. 1**).[1–3]

Upper Extremity

The most common levels of amputations for the upper limb are the transradial (TR) (below elbow, BE) and the transhumeral (TH) (above elbow, AE).

Lower Extremity

The most common levels of amputations for the lower limb are the transtibial (TT) (below knee, BK) and the transfemoral (TF) (above knee, AK).

Bilateral Amputees

For the bilateral lower limb amputee, energy expenditure becomes a major consideration in how functional and compliant the amputee is with prosthetics in comparison

[a] Amputee Services of America, 1601 East 19th Avenue, Suite 3200, Denver, CO 80218, USA; [b] Amputee Program, TIRR/Memorial Hermann Hospital, Houston, TX, USA; [c] Department of Physical Medicine and Rehabilitation, University of Texas Medical School, Houston, TX, USA; [d] Department of Orthopedic Surgery, University of Texas Medical School, Houston, TX, USA
* Corresponding author.
E-mail address: skipdoc3@gmail.com

Phys Med Rehabil Clin N Am 25 (2014) 199–212
http://dx.doi.org/10.1016/j.pmr.2013.09.011
1047-9651/14/$ – see front matter © 2014 Elsevier Inc. All rights reserved.

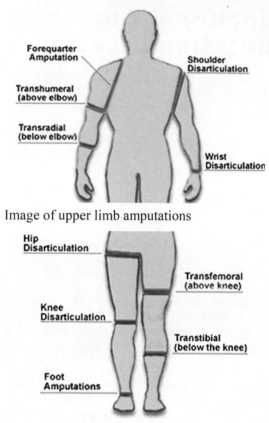

Image of upper limb amputations

Image of lower limb amputations

Fig. 1. Levels of limb amputations.

with mobility with a wheelchair. The bilateral lower limb amputee at the above-knee level is less likely to wear prosthetics, whereas the bilateral upper limb amputee is more likely to rely on prostheses in order to be more functionally independent.

REHABILITATION TEAM

Ideal outcomes for the amputee are best achieved by a multidisciplinary team including physicians, nurses, physical and occupational therapists, prosthetists, psychologists, vocational counselors, and social workers. Returning to independence and the highest level of function is the goal of the rehabilitation team. It is crucial for the team to identify issues such as pain, depression, and acceptance of changes experienced by the patient and his or her level of disability as a result of the amputation. Adapting to the use of a prosthesis is best accomplished by the team identifying and addressing potential barriers to wearing and using a prosthesis effectively.

PROSTHETIC CANDIDACY

Multiple factors that must be considered in determining whether a patient is an appropriate candidate for a prosthesis include cardiovascular endurance, level of amputation, cognitive ability, mobility goals, and comorbidities. For an upper extremity amputee, especially a unilateral amputee, depending on the timing of fitting a prosthesis one may be more functional without a cumbersome prosthesis. Others use their prosthesis only for a few hours a day as a tool to assist with certain activities. Early fitting for an upper limb amputation is essential because acceptance and compliance of wearing a prosthesis declines significantly after the third postoperative month. The Atkins Prosthetic Functional Adaptation Rating Scale rates compliance of using the prosthesis and how the prosthesis is used for bimanual tasks, and gross and fine motor tasks.

Atkins Prosthetic Functional Adaptation Rating Scale

100%: Wearing all day, using well in bilateral tasks, incorporating well in body scheme

75%: Wearing all day, using in gross and fine motor tasks

50%: Wearing all day, primarily for cosmetic reasons, using in gross motor tasks

0%: Not wearing or using the prosthesis; unilaterally independent

Lower extremity prostheses are more likely than upper extremity prostheses to be accepted, whereby appearance is often a factor. Function is more difficult to achieve with an upper limb prosthesis. Patients should be fitted within the first 3 months after an amputation to ensure the best acceptance rate of wearing a prosthesis, otherwise they tend to learn to accomplish tasks without the need of a prosthesis. Often patients require training for a new occupation that does not require using adaptive equipment. Driving should be achievable. Bilateral amputees are more likely than unilateral amputees to wear prostheses.

For lower limb amputees who may be bed bound or at a wheelchair level, especially for an AK, a prosthesis would not add any benefit for mobility goals, meaning that a prosthesis would not assist in transfers and only add weight and a cumbersome contraption. In this case the patient should focus on strengthening the sound limb and learning to transfer with a sliding board or walker. For a BK that is K1, a prosthesis may be helpful for transfers but ambulation may not be a realistic goal; for an AK transfers will not be enhanced or assisted with a prosthesis, and these patients transfer better with only an assistive device such as a sliding board or walker.

Energy expenditure and requirements increase significantly after an amputation, and are directly related to the length or level of amputation: the higher or more proximal the level of amputation, the more energy is required to ambulate with a prosthesis. Bilateral amputees have the highest energy requirement; in these cases, a wheelchair provides a faster and more effective mode of mobility.

Etiology also plays a role in the amount of energy that is expended in amputees. For amputations that occur from trauma, patients are often younger and healthier so their baseline level of activity is higher and can compensate better, reducing the amount of energy required to use their prosthesis. For amputations that occur from vascular disease, the baseline level of activity is typically much lower and, therefore, the energy requirement is often higher because these patients do not compensate as well from an endurance and cardiovascular standpoint (**Table 1**).

The Centers for Medicare and Medicaid (CMS) has devised a system to assign a potential level of ambulation function, called the K-level, which is determined by a physician and defines which prosthetic components are appropriate for that patient. The range is from 0 to 4, with K0 not being prosthetic candidates because they do not have the ability to ambulate or transfer with a prosthesis, whereas a K4 is a child or highly active adult. A K3-level amputee qualifies for energy-storing feet and higher-level knee units including pneumatic, hydraulic, or microprocessor knees (**Table 2**).

CMS requires the physician to document many items in the medical record to justify providing a prosthesis to a Medicare beneficiary. For specific documentation

Table 1
Energy requirements for types of amputation

Level of Amputation	Increased Energy Expenditure Above Normal (%)
Transtibial	20–25
Bilateral transtibial	41
Transfemoral	60–70
Transtibial/transfemoral	118
Bilateral transfemoral	>200

Data from Cuccurullo SJ. Physical medicine and rehabilitation board review. New York: Demos Medical Publishing; 2004; with permission.

requirements, a recommended template is currently being discussed to establish what information is needed in the physician's note. The required information is listed in the Physician Clinic Checklist (Appendix 1). Key objective outcome measures are used to identify the potential of a patient, which are addressed in an article by Heinemann and colleagues elsewhere in this issue. Some suggested measures include the following.

Objective Measures
- The amputee mobility predictor
- 6-minute walk test
- Timed Up and Go (TUG) test

Subjectively physicians can determine the patient's potential by clinical observation and/or using patient questionnaires.

Subjective Measures
- Locomotor Capabilities Index
- Activities-specific Balance Confidence (ABC) Scale

Table 2
K-level modifiers for Centers for Medicare and Medicaid Services (CMS)

K-Level 0	Does not have the ability or potential to ambulate or transfer safely with or without assistance, and a prosthesis does not enhance quality of life or mobility
K-Level 1	Has the ability or potential to use a prosthesis for transfers or ambulation in level surfaces at a fixed cadence. Typical of the limited and unlimited household ambulator
K-Level 2	Has the ability or potential for ambulation with the ability to transverse low-level environmental barriers such as curbs, stairs, or uneven surfaces. Typical of the limited community ambulator
K-Level 3	Has the ability or potential for ambulation with variable cadence. Typical of the community ambulator who has the ability to transverse most environmental barriers and may have vocational, therapeutic, or exercise activity that demands prosthetic use beyond simple locomotion
K-Level 4	Has the ability or potential for prosthetic ambulation that exceeds basic ambulation skills, exhibiting high impact, stress, or energy levels. Typical of the prosthetic demands of the child, active adult, or athlete

K is an arbitrary letter assigned by the Health Care Financing Administration to this classification system.

Adapted from Gailey RS, Roach KE, Applegate EB, et al. The amputee mobility predictor: an instrument to assess determinants of the lower-limb amputee's ability to ambulate. Arch Phys Med Rehabil 2002;83:613–62; with permission.

- Socket Fit Comfort Score
- Western Ontario and McMaster Universities Osteoarthritis Index (WOMAC)
- Oswestry Disability Questionnaire

Medical Record Documentation Required by CMS
See the Physician Clinic Checklist in Appendix 1.

Prosthetic fitting usually can be done within the first 3 to 6 weeks postoperatively with a preparatory or provisional prosthesis, with a definitive prosthesis at 6 to 8 months; a definitive prosthesis can eliminate the need for a preparatory one if aggressive shrinking is done in the first few weeks after sutures are removed. After continued shrinking occurs in the first year to 18 months, only replacement of the socket may be needed.

PHYSICAL THERAPY

Training begins with wound care, desensitization, stump shrinking, prevention of contractures (knee for BK, hip for AK), maintaining range of motion of the joints, and mastery of weight shifting and balance activities. A program of progressive ambulation begins on the parallel bars and progresses to the most independent level of ambulation possible, with or without gait aids.

Preprosthetic therapy should begin with a focus on transfers, bed mobility, wheelchair skills, and patient and family teaching. Maintaining or improving cardiovascular endurance with physical conditioning can be accomplished with wheelchair propulsion and single-limb ambulation with an assistive device or gait aid, lower limb strengthening, and upper limb ergometer for good upper body strength. Education on shrinking and shaping of the limb is also critical in maximizing the timing of the socket casting.

Prosthetic training begins with donning and doffing the prosthesis, education of sock management, skin evaluation, and establishment of a progressive prosthetic wearing schedule for wearing tolerance of the prosthesis; this process begins with 15 to 20 minutes' wear before removal to perform skin checks, followed by a gradual increase in the time worn until the amputee can wear the prosthesis full time, which will take several weeks.

Gait training with the prosthesis includes gaining knee stability, equal step lengths, and avoiding lateral trunk bending. After mastering ambulation of flat level surfaces, techniques are followed for managing uneven terrain, stairs, ramps, curbs, falling and getting up off the ground, then advancing from a walker to less cumbersome aids.

Once the amputee demonstrates safe ambulation and can ensure skin checks of the residual limb, he or she can take the prosthesis home.[4] A majority (97%) of all traumatic amputees were ambulating with a prosthesis at 3 months.[5] For dysvascular amputations, at a TT level, 78% of the patients wore a prosthesis, whereas only 57% of patients at a TF level wore a prosthesis (Physician Check list, Scientific & Medical Advisory Committee of the Amputee Coalition of America, Unpublished data).[6,7]

Therapy should also include driving, and getting in and out of a vehicle. Wheelchair assessment is also important as a backup mode of mobility or community mobility, whether amputees are to use a prosthesis or not. Custom chairs are lightweight, with rear wheels set posteriorly and antitippers.

OCCUPATIONAL THERAPY

Training is focused on donning and doffing the prosthesis, adjusting the number of sock plies, cleaning and caring for the residual limb and prosthesis, operating the terminal device with grasping and releasing objects, transferring objects, and positioning of the terminal device for functional activities. Amputation results in a loss of body symmetry and requires therapy to focus on rebalancing, and observing and correcting static postures and muscle memory to relearn correct postures. Repetitive tasks for strengthening, fine motor skills, and gross motor skills are part of the process. Specific movements necessary to control a prosthesis such as scapular abduction, humeral flexion, shoulder depression, extension and abduction, and chest expansion are also primary therapy goals. For the BE amputee the maintenance of range of motion of the elbow in flexion, extension, pronation, and supination is important for prosthetic use.

Evaluation of durable medical equipment for assistive and adaptive devices (reachers, long handles, sponges, shoehorns, dressing sticks, sock aids, long-handled mirrors) is necessary in addition to assessing the patient's home environment to maximize independence and safety. Most activities of daily living (ADLs) such as dressing, grooming, eating, and writing activities can be accomplished with one hand. The prosthesis can be helpful in managing zippers, donning socks and shoes, squeezing toothpaste onto the toothbrush, cutting meat (with an assistive device such as a rocker knife), and cutting paper with scissors.

ADLs, homemaking, and occupational and recreational activities are crucial to the amputee gaining functional independence. If the amputation has occurred on the dominant limb or if the amputee has bilateral limbs amputated, occupational therapy should focus on shirt buttoning, belt buckling, and toileting, as well as hand-dominance training for writing and keyboarding in the case of losing a dominant limb. For the bilateral amputee, foot skills should be a focus.[4]

PSYCHOLOGICAL THERAPY

Psychological assessment and identifying goals are key to understanding patients' expectations of what they can accomplish or in what phase of recovery they are. Describing the rehabilitation process to the patient can often be helpful in alleviating their concerns about leading a useful and independent life. Limb loss has been akin to a death, and the patient often goes through the stages of grief associated with loss. Fear, denial, anger, depression, and altered self-image are all psychological emotions that usually occur after an amputation and can affect interpersonal relationships, careers, and stresses of daily living. A psychologist can be effective in assisting the patient through this process and societal reintegration. A visitation by a certified peer visitor can also assist in this process.

VOCATIONAL REHABILITATION

Returning to work and school should be a main focus for recovery and rehabilitation of amputees. Employment is often essential for well-being, social reintegration, and a stable income. Adapting to the workplace and to any limitations imposed by the amputation is essential. Success in job integration is associated with younger age, higher education level, and wearing a more comfortable prosthesis. The patient may need to change to a physically less demanding type of work or undergo vocational training if unable to return to his or her prior job function with minimal dependence on assistive devices or adaptive equipment.

Timing for return to work and work capabilities are not well documented in the literature, nor tested in the workplace, for persons with amputations at specific levels. In addition, it is not uncommon for an amputee's personal physician to not understand what the expected capabilities would be for a particular level of amputation. For this reason, an experienced amputation rehabilitation physician should be involved in the decision to return to work, what work duties could be expected to be performed, and what specific work restrictions should apply for the individual.

If vocational services are considered useful for evaluation, further education, work-site modification, or job retraining, a referral to this service should be made. If vocational rehabilitation is not an entitlement of the workers' compensation law in a particular state, the state vocational rehabilitation agency should be approached to take an application for services.

In general, anyone of working age who has sustained a single amputation should be able to return to productive employment following amputation rehabilitation. If there are associated problems, this may not be possible. Even many bilateral amputees can be expected to return to work with modified duties or a modified work site.[8] An issue to be avoided is the functional capacity evaluation (FCE). Often the evaluator does not understand what the expected function of the worker should be, either with or without the use of a prosthesis. Moreover, the FCE should only be performed when the amputee has been conditioned to perform the tasks of the FCE and has full functional use of the prosthesis.

IDEAL OUTCOMES OF UPPER EXTREMITY AMPUTATION
Prosthesis Recommended:
    TR
        Body power
        External power
    TH
        Body power
        External power

The prosthesis is a tool in that it helps the single-limb amputee and the sound limb function as the dominant limb for all activities performed, regardless of prior hand dominance; therefore, change in hand dominance for writing and keyboarding is an imperative part of the process of rehabilitative therapy.

Ideally upper limb unilateral TR and TH amputees should be able to accomplish the following:

- Donning and doffing the prosthesis; wearing it during all waking hours, and using it for bimanual activities for at least 25% of manual activities
- Can perform one-handed activities including using a button hook
- Evaluated for adaptive equipment for ADLs
- Independent with basic ADLs
  - Personal needs: donning and doffing clothing, zippers, snaps, tying shoe laces with one hand, using a button hook; set time on watch/clock
  - Eating procedures: cutting meat (often with a rocker knife), opening milk carton
  - General household procedures: opening door knobs, phone use, writing, washing dishes, drying dishes with towel, use of tools such as hammer, tape measure
  - Meal preparation: cook, serve, and clean up using adaptive aids
  - Home repair: handling groceries, cleaning, minor plumbing
  - Child and pet care: diapering, holding, bathing, and feeding
  - Shopping: grocery and checkout process
  - Yard work: shovels, racks, mower
- Writing legibly with remaining hand; switch of dominance if necessary

- Driving and car procedure operations: assessment and training with modifications to vehicle (spinner knob) so as to operate/drive, open and close doors/trunk/hood
- Recreational and sports: training with terminal device depending on activity
- Returning to work: possible vocations include carpentry, auto repair; vocational training for work-related tasks may be required

Ideally bilateral upper limb amputees require a prosthesis to accomplish tasks.

- Donning and doffing the prosthesis with a dressing tree (requires setup)
- Evaluated for adaptive equipment for ADLs
- May require some caregiver assistance with basic ADLs
  - Personal needs: donning and doffing clothing
  - Eating procedures: cutting meat (often with a rocker knife), opening milk carton
  - General household procedures: opening door knobs, phone use, writing, washing dishes, drying dishes with towel, use of tools such as hammer, tape measure
  - Meal preparation: cook, serve, and clean up using adaptive aids
  - Child and pet care: diapering, holding, bathing, and feeding
  - Shopping: grocery and checkout process
  - Yard work: shovels, racks, mower
- Driving and car procedure operations: assessment and training with modifications to vehicle to operate/drive, open and close doors/trunk/hood
- Returning to work: vocational training for work-related tasks may be required depending on prior job function

IDEAL OUTCOMES OF LOWER EXTREMITY AMPUTATION

TT prosthesis recommended: provisional and definitive.

- Ambulation with prosthesis on level and uneven surfaces, stairs, ramps, and curbs
- Ambulation with minimal or no gait aids
- Independent with dressing
- Independent in donning and doffing prosthesis
- Independent in stump wrapping or applying a shrinker
- Able to drive
- Can participate in shopping activities
- Has returned to previous work, with or without modifications
- Can stand for up to 2 continuous hours
- Can sit for up to 2 continuous hours
- Can arise from the kneeling position
- Comfortable with falling techniques and can arise from the floor
- Can hunt, fish, run, bicycle (if part of previous lifestyle)
- Knows how to purchase properly fitting footwear for the remaining foot
- Knows proper skin and nail care for remaining foot
- Can safely perform aerobic conditioning program
- Climbs stairs foot over foot

TF prosthesis recommended: provisional and definitive.

- Ambulation with prosthesis on level and uneven surfaces, stairs, ramps, and curbs
- Ambulation with minimal or no gait aids
- Independent with dressing

- Independent in donning and doffing prosthesis
- Independent in stump wrapping or applying a shrinker
- Able to drive
- Can participate in shopping activities
- Has returned to previous work, with or without modifications
- Can stand for up to 2 continuous hours
- Can sit for up to 2 continuous hours
- Can arise from the kneeling position
- Comfortable with falling techniques and can arise from the floor
- Can hunt, fish, bicycle (if part of previous lifestyle)
- Knows how to purchase properly fitting footwear for the remaining foot
- Knows proper skin and nail care for remaining foot
- Can safely perform aerobic conditioning program
- Stairs are generally climbed one at a time
- Can run (if amputee desires, has adequate cardiopulmonary reserve and residual limb length)
- Uses no more than a cane for ambulation

Bilateral amputees may find that the energy expenditure required to ambulate with prostheses is too great to comply with using them. Often a wheelchair is faster and more effective in mobility.

- Ambulation with prostheses on level and uneven surfaces, stairs, ramps, and curbs
- Ambulation with gait aids is often required
- Independent with dressing
- Independent in donning and doffing prosthesis
- Independent in stump wrapping or applying a shrinker
- Able to drive with hand controls
- Can participate in shopping activities
- Can return to previous work, with modifications
- Can sit for up to 2 continuous hours
- Can safely perform aerobic conditioning program, often with an ergometer hand cycle

MEASURABLE FUNCTIONAL OUTCOMES

Specific outcome measures are addressed in the article by Heinemann elsewhere in this issue.

SUMMARY

Understanding and educating patients on the ideal outcomes provides a goal-oriented rehabilitation plan after an amputation. Knowing what is achievable can make an overwhelming life-changing event into one that has a brighter outlook than was likely initially anticipated. As a physician who treats amputees, having this information provides a detailed prescriptive plan for the rehabilitation team to accomplish, thus allowing the amputee the best chance at achieving the ideal functional outcome.

REFERENCES

1. Sheehan T. Rehabilitation and prosthetic restoration in upper limb amputation. Braddom. p. 257–316.

2. Robert HM III, Esquenazi A. Follow-up, outcomes and long-term experiences in adults with upper extremity amputation; functional restoration of adults and children with upper extremity amputation. p. 327–36.
3. Cohen J, Edelstein J. Limb deficiency, medical aspects of disability. In: Flanagan S, Herbert H, Zaretsky Y, et al, editors. A handbook for the rehabilitation professional. 4th edition; 2011. p. 381–408.
4. Gitter A, Bosker G. Upper and lower extremity prosthetics. In: Frontera WR, editor. DeLisa's physical medicine and rehabilitation: principles and practice, two volume set (rehabilitation medicine). 2005. p. 1325–53.
5. MacKenzie EJ, Bosse MJ, Castillo RC, et al. Functional outcomes following trauma-related lower-limb amputation. J Bone Joint Surg Am 2004;86(8): 1636–45.
6. Fletcher DD, Andrew KL, Hallet JW, et al. Trends in rehabilitation after amputation for geriatric patients with vascular disease: implications for future health resource allocations. Arch Phys Med Rehabil 2002;83(10):1389–93.
7. Atkins DJ. Adult upper limb prosthetic training. In: Bowker JH, Micheal JW, editors. Altas of limb prosthetics: surgical, prosthetic, and rehabilitation principles. 2nd edition. St Louis (MO): Mosby; 1992. p. 275–84.
8. Meier RH. Life care planning for the amputee. In: Weed RO, Berens DE, editors. Life care planning and case management handbook (Chapter 12). 3rd edition. Boca Raton: CRC Press; 2010.

APPENDIX 1

Physician Clinic Documentation for Lower Limb Amputee Management and Care

Reason for visit/Chief Complaint:
- Prosthetic and rehabilitation evaluation
- Requesting new prosthesis or artificial limb
- Problem with prosthesis or artificial limb

Amputation History (History of Present Illness)

Etiology/Cause of Amputation
- Trauma ☐ Diabetes/Diabetic foot sore
- Infection ☐ Vascular Disease
- Cancer/Tumor ☐ Other:_____

Date of Amputation(s)
- _____

Amputation level
- Hip disarticulation
- Above knee (Trans-femoral)
- Below knee (Trans-tibia)
- Symes (Ankle disarticulation)
- Partial Foot
- Toes (s)

Prognosis of ambulation with Prosthesis
- Good ☐ Fair ☐ Poor
- Motivated to use/wear a prosthesis
- Wants therapy for prosthetic training
- Functional non-amputated limb(s)

Goals for using a prosthesis:
- Vocational requirement
- Athletic goals
- Basic locomotion

Past Medical/Surgical History: **Y** if patient has Diagnosis

Diabetes	Peripheral Vascular Disease
High Blood Pressure	Congestive Heart Failure
Chronic Lung Disease	Arthritis
Parkinson Disease	Peripheral Neuropathy
Chronic Pain	Dementia

Recent amputation complications _____
Past amputation complications: _____
Recent medication changes: _____
Planned surgical revision of amputation? **(Y/N)**

Social History:
# of Steps/stairs needed to navigate in home
Needs a caregiver to don/doff prosthesis? **(Y/N)**
Needs to navigate different level terrain? **(Y/N)**

Review of Systems: (Y if present)
Constitutional: Changes in weight of greater than 10 lbs?
Eyes: Poor vision limiting safe walking with prosthesis?
Resp: Supplemental oxygen is required?
Resp: Shortness of breath with activity?
CVS: Claudication present with ambulation?
MSK: Recent falls?
MSK: Chronic pain syndrome or phantom pain?
Neuro: Abnormal gait and balance?
Skin: Amputated limb skin breakdown?
Cognitive: Cognition impaired?

Endocrine: Uncontrolled diabetes?

Emotional: Non-treated Depression from limb loss?

Patient's Functional Status

CURRENT Activities of Daily Living (ADLs):

I = independent, **A** = assistance needed, **NA** = not applicable

Bathing   Toileting   Driving

Dressing (putting on socks, shirt/pants)

Transfers (getting up from a seated position)

MOBILITY STATUS

Assistive Devices **AD**: Rolling Walker **RW**, Cane **SPC**

Non-ambulatory: Wheelchair **WC,** Power Mobility Device **PMD**

Community ambulatory without limitations

Before amputation used an AD to walk? **Y/N**

Post-amputation, mobility device used? **RW, SPC, WC, PMD**

Has sufficient strength/endurance to use a prosthesis? **Y/N**

CURRENT FUNCTIONAL STATUS

Functional CMS Level:

- **K0** – Prosthesis not functional for activities
    Cosmetic only
- **K1** - Ability to transfer; household ambulation
- **K2** - Ability to ambulate short community distances
- **K3** - Ambulatory over all community distances
    Uses variable cadence
- **K4** - Abilities above normal ambulation,
    Recreational and sports

EXPECTED/POTENTIAL FUNCTIONAL STATUS

If different than current (Circle)

K0   K1   K2   K3   K4

Reach this K level in a reasonable amount of time? (Y/N)

Reason for the difference: _____

PROSTHESIS

Patient has a prosthesis? (Y/N)

Age of Prosthesis (in years)

Wearing time of prosthesis:

- Less than 4 hours per day
- 4 to 8 hours per day
- More than 8 hours per day
- Other: _____

Problems with current prosthesis: (Y/N)

Describe: _____

Can prosthetic components be replaced?_: (Y/N)

Describe: _____

Is a new prosthesis required? : (Y/N)

Reason: _____

Prescription: _____

_____

_____

_____

_____

_____

_____

Physical Exam: (Vital Signs)
Constitutional
     Height
     Weight
  Psychiatric:
- Normal mental status, judgment, insight
- Normal memory
- Other:_____
  Eyes:
- Normal visual acuity
- Blindness, severely decreased vision
  Respiratory
- 6-minute walk test: _____ft.
- Non-labored breath sounds
- Required oxygen
- Used accessory intercostal muscles
  Cardiovascular
- Regular rate and rhythm
- Jugular venous distention
- Lower extremity edema
- Other:_____
  Strength in upper extremities
- Normal 5/5
- Other:_____
  Strength in non-amputated limb
- Normal 5/5
- Other:_____
  Strength in residual limb
- Normal 5/5
- Other:_____ __
  Range of Motion
- Normal
- No contractures
- Other:_____
  Neurological
- Sensory intact
- Peripheral neuropathy
- Other:_____
  Balance and Coordination
- Normal
- Other:_____
  Transfers:
- Transfers independently from WC
- Transfers using a sliding board
- Unable to transfer (requires lift or assistance)
  Standing:
- Able to stand from a seated position
  Gait
- Non-ambulatory, Wheelchair
- Unassisted, Steady, Symmetric
- Assistive Device: _____

- Unsteady
- Antalgic

Stride length:
- ☐ Normal
- ☐ Wide based
- ☐ Narrow based

- Hip hike
- Truck lean   ☐ Circumduction
- Knee buckling   ☐ Drop foot

Current Status of Residual Limb
Length:
- Short
- Mid-level
- Long

Shape of Limb:
- Ready for prosthesis (Conical, Cylindrical)
- Needs shrinking and shaping (Bulbous)
- Prosthetic accommodations for (Bony Prominence, decreased soft tissue coverage)

Color of residual limb:
- Normal
- Other:_____

Temperature of residual limb:
- Normal, warm
- Other:_____

Skin Incision:
- Well healed
- Staples/Sutures
- Intact STSG (split thickness skin graft)
- Moist
- Necrotic
- Dry

Drainage:
- None
- Purulent drainage
- Serosanginous
- Serous

Physician Name: _____ Signature: _____ Date:_____ NPI: _____

Courtesy of Centers for Medicare and Medicaid Services, Baltimore, MD.

A Quote for the Conclusion of the Text

"To listen well is as powerful a means of communication as to talk well."
—John Marshall, 1755–1835, Fourth Chief Justice of the United States and one of the namesakes for Franklin and Marshall College, Lancaster, Pennsylvania

Phys Med Rehabil Clin N Am 25 (2014) 213
http://dx.doi.org/10.1016/j.pmr.2013.10.005
1047-9651/14/$ – see front matter © 2014 Published by Elsevier Inc.

pmr.theclinics.com

Index

Note: Page numbers of article titles are in **boldface** type.

Phys Med Rehabil Clin N Am 25 (2014) 215–228
http://dx.doi.org/10.1016/S1047-9651(13)00095-8
1047-9651/14/$ – see front matter © 2014 Elsevier Inc. All rights reserved.

Printed in Australia by Griffin Press
an Accredited ISO AS/NZS 14001:2004
Environmental Management System printer.